Cook Yourself Thin

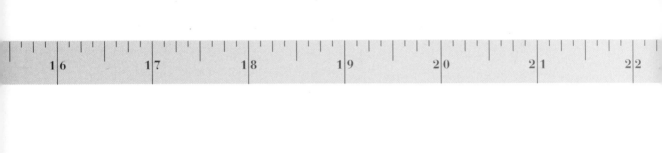

Cook Yourself
THIN

Skinny Meals You
Can Make in Minutes

voice
HYPERION   NEW YORK

Potential results will vary. Consult with your healthcare professional for health
and nutritional information and before undertaking any new diet.

Copyright © 2009 Lifetime Entertainment Services

Photography by Evan Sung

All rights reserved. No part of this book may be used or reproduced in any
manner whatsoever without the written permission of the Publisher. Printed
in the United States of America. For information address Hyperion, 114 Fifth
Avenue, New York, New York 10011.

Library of Congress Cataloging-in-Publication Data

Cook yourself thin : skinny meals you can make in minutes / Lifetime Television.
    p. cm.
  ISBN 978-1-4013-4113-8
  1. Cookery. 2. Low-fat diet—Recipes. 3. Low-calorie diet—Recipes.
I. Lifetime Television (Firm) II. Cook yourself thin (Television program)
  TX714.C65416 2009
  641.5'635—dc22   2009008165

Hyperion books are available for special promotions and premiums. For details
contact the HarperCollins Special Markets Department in the New York office
at 212-207-7528, fax 212-207-7222, or email spsales@harpercollins.com.

Packaged and Designed by Dolphin & Jones Book Packaging and Media

FIRST EDITION

10 9 8 7 6 5

Acknowledgments

The *Cook Yourself Thin* cookbook, like the television series, required the dedication and hard work of many people. From the Tiger Aspect UK team, where the show was created and originated, many thanks are due to: Andrew Zein, Managing Director, Jo McGrath, Head of Features, Jenny Spearing, and Elaine Foster, along with more help from London from Gordon Wise and Michael Joseph.

For the American version of the series and for this cookbook, enormous thanks to the Tiger Aspect USA/IMG team: Adam Steinman, VP of Development, Christine Connor, Executive Producer, Lauren Deen, Co-Executive Producer and in-house editor of the book, and the entire production staff and crew who enabled us to produce the book during the shooting of the television series.

A dedicated team of professionals worked tirelessly on the book and deserve enormous thanks: Evan Sung for the beautiful photography, Morgan Bennison for gorgeous food styling, Natasha Louise King, prop stylist extraordinaire, and Joe Delate for the colorful wardrobe, along with the editorial support of Diane Perez, Henry Tenney, Elizabeth Darst, Jessica Pantzer, Annie Petito, Lindsay Freed, Eddie Roche, Jennifer Weinberg, and Stephanie Lyness. On the business affairs and legal end, many thanks to the efforts of Peter Devita.

Hyperion has been an exceptional partner and we are grateful for the efforts of Ellen Archer and Barbara Jones, Voice Editorial Director, and our wonderful editor, Sarah Landis.

For Lifetime Television, special thanks for the creative vision and all-around support of Andrea Wong, JoAnn Alfano, Jessica Samet, Sandy Varo, Julie Stern, Linda Rein, Beck Sloca, and Doug Strasnick.

Contents

Sweets

Have your cake and eat it too!

This book will help you lose weight. But it's not a diet book. Think of it more as a guide to stop starving yourself and start loving food, because you really can lose the bulge and still indulge.

Cook Yourself Thin is for normal women, just like you. We know that you love to eat but we are realistic enough to know that you can't eat anything and everything and expect to look hot in a bikini. It was created for busy people, people like you, who are not prepared to give up social lives or favorite treats to become slaves to a strict diet. The CYT philosophy figures out the solutions, so you don't have to.

You may have tried most of the diets out there—and failed. And you're not the only one. One major weight-loss study has found that up to two-thirds of dieters put all the weight they lost back on within five years—and most end up even heavier! No matter what the diet, the study found, it's unlikely to lead to lasting weight loss.

Sure, you will lose weight if you follow a diet to the letter. But how many of us stay on a diet—is that any way to enjoy life? Most diet food tastes awful and the portions are tiny, which means you fall off the wagon in spectacular style. Then follows the guilt, shame, feeling bad about yourself, and the almost inevitable overeating. It's a bad cycle. It's no good for your mind, body, or soul.

You've probably gone to all sorts of lengths to feel thinner. We've all subjected ourselves to the grapefruit diets, Weight Watchers-style clubs, and years of yo-yo dieting. Some even flit from feast to famine, never quite finding a happy balance. And yet denial is the fastest way to find yourself up to your eyeballs in chocolate.

Quick fixes won't work and there's only one simple way to lose weight and keep it off without losing your mind: cook yourself thin.

Step Away from the Scales

The fact is, most of us don't need to change our eating habits completely. We just need to make smart but simple changes. Dieticians and nutritionists agree that low-fat, low-calorie cooking skills, along with a basic knowledge of food labels and portion sizes, are the key to keeping slim. It has been suggested that consuming just 100 fewer calories a day (about one cookie's worth) will prevent the average yearly weight gain of 2 pounds. That's not exactly starving yourself.

Another study showed that most of us are used to eating just that little bit too much. It found that women who consumed 800 fewer calories a day than normal felt just as full and satisfied. They did it by making *small* changes—for example, skim milk instead of whole, eating half as much cheese, more vegetables, and less fat overall. Small changes like these are easier to stick to and harder to go back on. But they add up to a significant drop in calories—and dress size.

The CYT approach takes a positive attitude toward food. No denial or guilt—just the promise of mouthwatering delights instead of dull food. In this book, you'll be able to quickly and easily figure out how and why you're consuming a few too many calories, and learn the secret to cutting down without losing out. CYT takes up the challenge and does all the homework to make it easy for you. You don't have to become a culinary queen, you just need to cook more and cook *smarter.*

Here are tried, tested, and tasted favorite recipes with all the cheats, tips, tricks, and swaps worked out to make your calories vanish into thin air. At *Cook Yourself Thin* we have really high standards, so you won't find any recipe or suggestion that we're not convinced is better than the calorie-laden original. We all love a challenge, and we've created recipes that use flavors and ingredients that will leave you speechless. All it takes is a little effort and you can learn to re-create your beloved takeout food, comfort meals, snacks and desserts. And that's all there is to it: no weird foods or diet supplements, no denial, no sweaty exercise regime—just flavor, satisfaction, and no more clothes that just fit; they flaunt your better body.

> So get ready to Cook Yourself Thin!

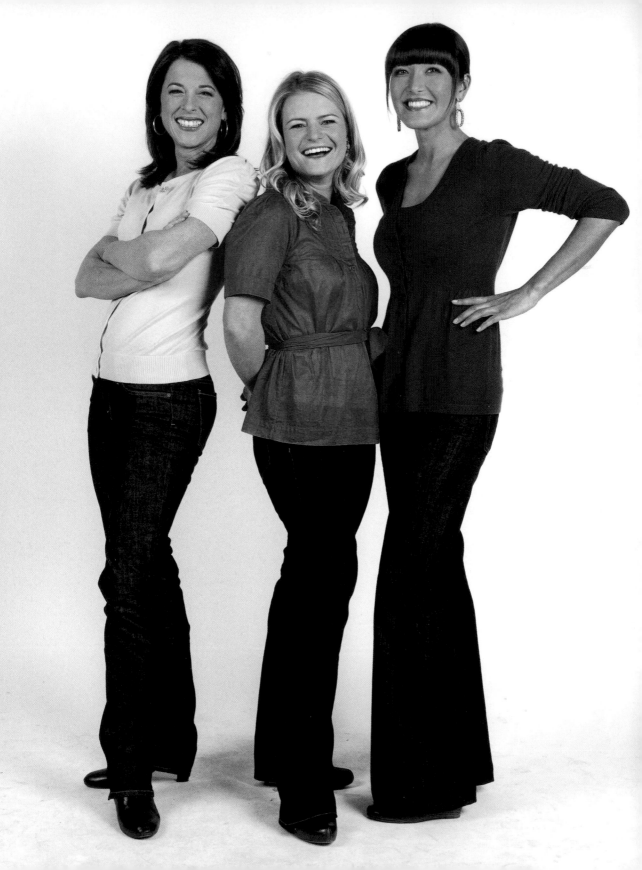

Meet the
Cook Yourself Thin Team

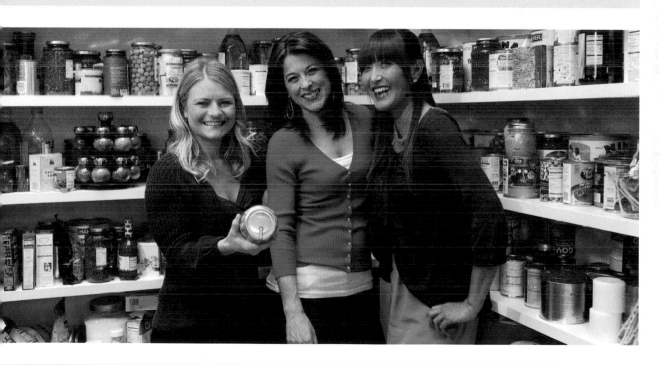

Harry Eastwood

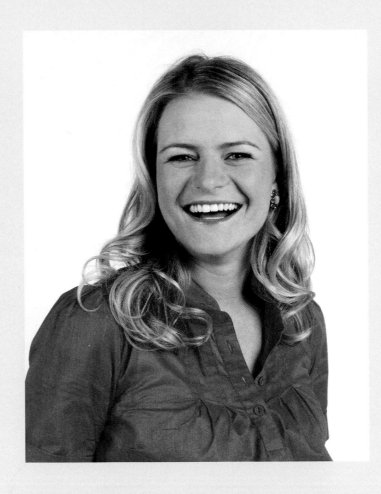

Harry has lived in Qatar, France, and London, as well as Sydney for a spell, and has been exposed to a colorful mix of cuisines and cultures. She loves making food from scratch and inventing new dishes. For the past seven years, she's worked as both a food stylist and writer, with a flair for sourcing the most beautiful ingredients around and interpreting every recipe under the sun. She is also a co-host of the original, British hit version of *Cook Yourself Thin*.

Just to prove that appearances can be deceiving, Harry is into pink, sparkly earrings, all things pretty, and oh, butchery. That's right, she loves to prepare meat from field to plate so she knows exactly where her dishes have come from and what's gone into them. And forget fashion labels, Harry's into food labels—the higher quality the ingredients, the better. But censoring her ingredients is as far as food restrictions go. Her philosophy is that if you crave something, it usually means your body (and soul) deserves it. She genuinely considers chocolate to be good for the soul and feels that it completes a meal the way a period completes a sentence.

It'll come as no surprise, then, that Harry most definitely does not believe in restrictive diets. Food, she says, has been the joyful background to her life and learning to cook is the best weight-loss tool there is.

Candice Kumai

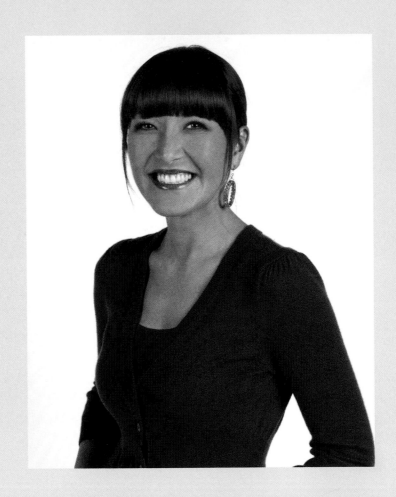

Candice is from San Diego and grew up living the life of a true California girl—surfing, sunshine, hanging at the beach, and having fun. As a teen, she became a fashion model and spent eight years traveling the nation and the world on assignments. But despite the glamour of modeling, she always felt deep down that her true calling in life was cooking.

Her mother, a graduate of Tokyo Gakugei University, was born in southern Japan and her father is a Naval veteran of Polish-American descent. She learned the essentials of those culinary traditions from her mother and grandmothers. After earning a bachelor's degree she decided to pursue cooking professionally and did so at the prestigious Le Cordon Bleu California School of Culinary Arts Program, where she won honors as "Top of the Class," President's List, and Dean's List.

Candice has since cooked at several well-respected restaurants in Los Angeles and Orange County, such as the Ritz Carlton Laguna Niguel, and she worked for Chef Wolfgang Puck. She has appeared on Bravo's *Top Chef*, where her upbeat personality, charm, and cooking talents won her many fans. Her dream is to follow in the footsteps of her idols Julia Child and Martha Stewart and become the food/lifestyle guru of her generation. She brings as much passion and flair to cooking as she does to everything in life—her ideal is to bring together all of the things she loves: fashion, friends, and great food.

Allison Fishman

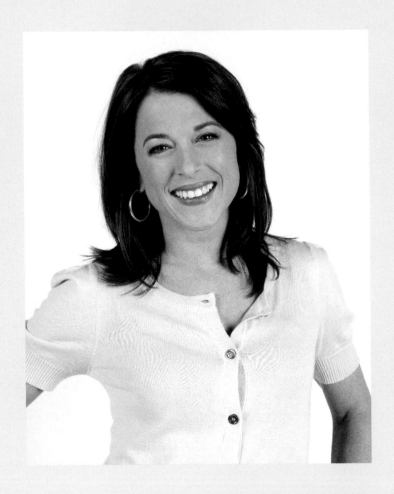

$\mathcal{Allison}$ is passionate about food—not just cooking and eating it, but also writing about and studying it. She understands the joy and pleasure of food from every angle—as an academic, writer, trained chef, and food lover.

To share this passion she created a cooking school called The Wooden Spoon, where she and her team of instructors come to people's homes, demonstrating for them the techniques and deliciousness of home cooking. She loves being able to help people become excited about food and confident and creative in their own kitchens.

She has lent her talents as a recipe developer and food stylist to various magazines and television projects, including Martha Stewart, the Food Network, *Real Simple*, and *Glamour* magazines. As a former co-host of TLC's *Home Made Simple*, Allison traveled the country showing families how to cook confidently in their own kitchens.

Allison has a B.S. in human development and family studies from Cornell University, and a culinary degree from the Institute for Culinary Education. She's currently pursuing a master's degree in food studies from New York University, just a subway stop away from her home in Brooklyn.

Philosophy

What's Your Eater ID?

Take our fast quiz to identify the obstacles that trip you up when it comes to eating. Put this together with what you've learned from your food diary, and you'll know what kind of eater you are and where to cut the calories for super-fast results. Ready?

A Quick Quiz

What are your dieting downfalls? Choose the answer that best matches you.

What's in your fridge right now?

A. Half a bottle of diet soda, a takeout container, and something unidentifiable with green stuff growing on it

B. A half-eaten giant slab of chocolate, a slice of pie, and peanut butter

C. Some smoked salmon, a few eggs, a chilled bottle of vodka

D. Milk, cheese, leftover meatloaf

What would your desert-island dish be?

A. General Tso's chicken

B. Chocolate mousse cake

C. Since I'd be near the ocean, oysters and champagne

D. Pot roast with mashed potatoes

Which of these diets have you tried?

A. Low-fat

B. You name it

C. Carb-free

D. I've never dieted

What's your ideal dinner date?

A. Ordering Asian and cozying up on the couch

B. Having giant sundaes at an ice-cream parlor

C. Going out to the hot new restaurant in town

D. Hamburger and fries at a bar

When was the last time you ordered takeout?

A. About 12 hours ago

B. Besides taking the ice cream from the freezer?

C. When I had some friends over last night

D. Rarely—I'd rather cook myself

When's the last time you skipped a meal?

A. I skip breakfast but always eat at night, even if it's late
B. Sometimes I go right to dessert
C. If I'm out, I'll skip dinner
D. When I had the stomach flu in 1998

Your favorite drink?

A. A double latte
B. Hot chocolate with mini-marshmallows
C. Champagne, what else?
D. Diet soda

You've been dumped. What do you do?

A. Have my friends over for DVDs and popcorn
B. Stay in bed with a tub of ice cream
C. Hit the town and flirt up a storm
D. Cook a big meal—it helps me relax

What kind of exercise do you get?

A. Running out the door to work
B. Hmm, exercise, yes, I should...
C. I'm a gym rat—I take pride in my muscles
D. I love long walks.

Favorite veggies?

A. French fries
B. Broccoli
C. Corn on the cob
D. Butternut squash

You and your kitchen—best friend or feared enemy?

A. I store my sweaters in the stove like Carrie
B. We're like friends who have less in common these days
C. We don't spend much time together
D. We're soul mates

What item defines your kitchen?

A. An overflowing garbage can
B. My heart-shaped cookie cutters
C. A wok—for quick meals before I go out
D. A giant casserole dish

What's the ideal way to end a meal?

A. Going to bed
B. Ice cream, of course
C. Dancing at my favorite club
D. Cheese tray

What's your meal to impress a new man?

A. I'd buy fancy prepared gourmet meals and hide the packages
B. Love me, love my tiramisu
C. As if! He's taking me to dinner!
D. A perfect steak and apple pie for dessert

What do you eat when you're starving?

A. A bag of potato chips
B. I'm never starving, I always keep chocolate nearby
C. Fancy hors d'oeuvres
D. Peanut butter and jelly

How do you feel about diets?

A. I should eat less junk, but I don't have time to cook
B. If I'm not supposed to eat it, I want it desperately
C. If I've overeaten, I just eat less for a few days
D. Everything in moderation—but moderation is tricky to stick with

How Did You Score?

Mostly A's
You're an ON-THE-RUN EATER

You have the local Chinese, fried chicken, and pizza places on speed dial. And they probably know your name and order before you've even said hello. Lunchtime consists of whatever salad bar the nearest deli has to offer, and just about everything else you eat is chow on the run. We get it—you're busy. But trust us, you'll feel a lot less frantic and stressed (and bloated) if you brave the kitchen every once in a while. Cooking doesn't have to be hard, as you'll see from our recipes. And you'll find that some of your favorite takeout meals can be created at a fraction of the cost, in the same amount of time it takes for them to be delivered. And—most important—with nothing close to the calories and fat you're currently consuming.

Mostly B's
You're a SUGAR FIEND

You were born with a spoonful of sugar in your mouth. You'd happily give up takeout food, frozen dinners, and all sorts of junk food as long as you didn't have to sacrifice your daily sweet treats. There's always something chocolaty in your cupboard, in your glove compartment, in your purse, and in your desk at work—just in case. And if you can't finish a meal with something sweet, you almost feel a panic attack coming on. Although you know you have an "issue" with sugary foods, you feel powerless to resist. And that's why we've worked out some super-rich decadent treats that will give you your sugar high, without the guilt-ridden low. With a teensy bit of effort, you can have your cake and eat it too.

Mostly C's
You're a **YO-YO DIETER**

Your appearance is important to you, so you make more effort than most not to totally pig out at mealtimes. Problem is, your self-restraint is so good you often skip meals altogether. Health aside, this ultimately has the effect of making your body think it's starving, so it'll hold onto any fat stores you have. Not a good idea. Time is also an issue for you. You often head out for drinks straight from work, and unless food is available, you'll forget all about it and fill up on alcoholic empty calories. And watch out—because alcohol is packed with calories. What, you didn't know that? We're not suggesting you stop your social life and stay in—heaven forbid! But try some of our smart calorie swaps and super-fast meal ideas and you'll soon find fitting into your skinny jeans is much easier.

Mostly D's
You're a **COMFORT FOOD CRAVER**

You love food and home-cooked meals. Some of your favorite recipes have been in your family for years, and just the smell of them makes you feel safe and happy. You're also a modern foodie and love to sample the latest bistro. You have a pretty good idea about nutrition and how to create a flavorful, satisfying meal, but your enthusiasm for eating means portion control doesn't enter your mind. Some of your cooking methods and ingredients are as antiquated as your recipes (it *is* possible to make mashed potatoes without a stick of butter and cream, you know). Fortunately, while our recipes cut down on calories, they never compromise on taste or comfort. Open your mind to some new ingredients and techniques, and you can feel cozy without looking like a plush teddy bear.

So You Want to Drop a Dress Size?

Join the club! Most women say they'd be happier if they could buy their jeans a size smaller, spare the horror of suck-it-all-in spandex supports, and drop that extra 10 pounds they've been toting around since the beginning of the holidays—circa 2001.

Contrary to media reports we're not all obese. Nor, thank goodness, are we all a size 2. The average dress size in the United States is 12. Only 33 percent of women are classified as obese, but 62 percent are overweight (ouch!), so we do need to control our eating. But despite the newspaper headlines, for most of us it's not about a total body transformation—we'd just like to get a little closer to our "happy weight" and feel healthy and attractive.

It's a reasonable goal, so why does it seem so hard to achieve? Because, girls, we're kidding ourselves. All too easily we buy into the diet industry propaganda that tells us all our problems will be solved if we just cut out X or supplement with Y. We want to believe that weight-loss success comes only in the form of denying ourselves all things pleasurable. And when the inevitable happens and we fall off the diet wagon, we have the perfect excuse to decide that losing weight is impossible for us, and just give up.

The fact is, whether you think you're super-healthy and restrained or you acknowledge that your dietary halo needs a good polish, you—like all of us in the past—have probably been deluding yourself. What you think of as an occasional habit may well have become a permanent fixture in your life. That large latte and blueberry muffin you blithely scarf down most mornings? That's 765 calories every day. Read it and weep. The bacon sandwich and can of Coke that never fails to cure your hangover—540 calories. The Friday night pizza—a whopping 1,000 calories. Fine from time to time, but if these are a regular part of your diet, it's no wonder you think those skinny jeans have shrunk.

You don't have to consume junk food around the clock to put on weight. There are certain foods that are just too darn delish and tempting to resist, and the truth is you probably give in to them just a little more often than you admit to yourself. *Cook Yourself Thin* doesn't want you to resist them either, just keep reading so you can cook or prepare many of them in a way that is far more delicious than the store-bought options, with a fraction of the calories.

Fact

Contrary to media reports, we're not all obese. Nor, thank goodness, a size 2. The average dress size in the United States is 12.

All we ask of you is a little effort in the kitchen and some good old-fashioned honesty. Brace yourself—you'll need to keep a food diary for a week. But don't panic. This is not going to be one of those boring, document-keeping diets. And it's the last bit of hard work you'll need to do.

So grab a notebook that's small and stylish enough that you won't mind carrying it around with you all week. Ditto a cool pen. Give yourself a couple of pages for each day and write the name of the day across the top of the page. Then, from the moment you get up until the minute you hit the pillow at night, record every last morsel of food or sip of liquid that passes your lips. This is super important—because, more often than not, it's our more unconscious habits that get us into trouble. So that handful of tortilla chips at a cocktail party, the tiny slice of cake you had at a co-worker's birthday party, the little pieces of cheese you slice off every time you go to the fridge—they all count, because the devil is in the details.

Be prepared to finish up with really long lists every day. This is normal. To help you get started, here's an example:

MORNING
- Glass of orange juice
- Black coffee
- 2 slices of thick white toast with butter
- Banana
- Large latte with a shot of syrup
- Half a bag of licorice

AFTERNOON
- Chicken burger on a bun with mayo, salad with French dressing, French fries and ketchup
- 2 Diet Cokes
- 2 small cookies
- A handful of chocolate chips

EVENING
- Half a large bag of tortilla chips
- Half a container of hummus
- One frozen lasagna dinner
- 2 glasses of white wine
- Cup of decaf espresso
- Cup of rice pudding
- Chocolate chip cookie

When your diary is complete, give yourself half an hour to sit down and analyze it. Remember, this isn't an exercise in feeling bad about yourself. On the contrary, it's empowering. It's the perfect way to identify what your tastes and personal must-haves are when it comes to food and how to make sure you still satisfy that culinary lust as you shrink in size.

There's no magic scientific formula for the analysis—but a few different-colored highlighter pens might come in handy. We just want you to scan your lists for patterns. These might be easy to spot (half a tub of ice cream, 9 p.m. weekdays) or less obvious (like the fact that you eat more when you're cooking for your guy). Make a note of anything that occurs to you. It might be useful to highlight these and then add up the following:

- Any foods or drinks that show up every day
- All alcoholic drinks
- All non-diet carbonated drinks
- All food bought and eaten on the run (like a sandwich)
- All takeout meals
- All meals out
- Sweet snacks
- Savory/salty snacks
- Pig-out sessions

Hopefully, you'll see one or two patterns emerge from this process. You might discover that you tend to "graze" all day long, which can be perfectly fine if that means fruit for snacks and small portions at mealtimes, but start adding hunks of cheese and endless bags of chips to three average meals a day and you can quickly see why the calories might be adding up. Or maybe you've gotten into the habit of grabbing a candy bar every day at the same time. It's a pick-me-up you now feel you couldn't do without, but once you try the sinfully good Mint Chocolate Cupcakes (page 210), you'll never look back. Many people eat pretty well during the week and then blow it all on the weekend on a few too many glasses of wine, takeout food, and massive brunches, while others are happy to spend time cooking wholesome meals during the weekend, but don't have the time during the week. In the next few pages, you'll pick up plenty of tips and tricks to help you pinpoint the easy changes you can make to cut your calories and start seeing the pounds drop off.

A Quick Guide to Calories

If you're female and you made it as far as your mid-teens without using the word "calorie," congratulations! There can't be too many body-conscious women out there who aren't familiar with the term. But do we really know what it means? Time for a quick lesson.

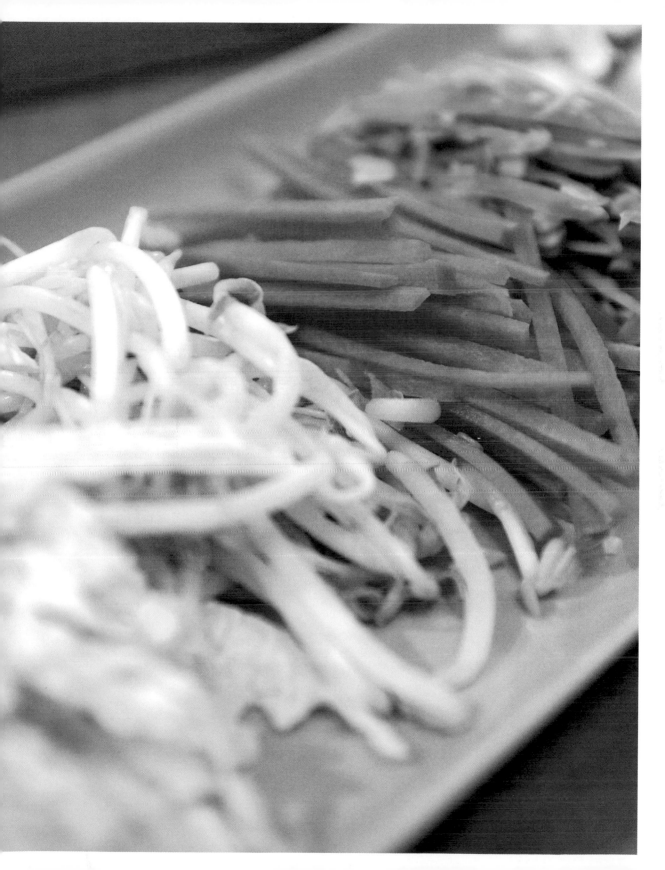

$\mathcal{A}$ calorie is basically a unit that measures how much energy your body is able to get from food. Different nutrients in food provide different amounts of calories: for example, fat gives you about 9 calories per gram, alcohol 7, while carbohydrates and protein yield about 4.

To find out how many calories a food contains, you can either consult our Calorie Guide (page 40) or check the nutritional information on the food label if it comes in a package. Remember to check the *number of servings* this refers to though. Most labels show nutritional information for one serving of the product. Even some seemingly tiny packages (like a small bag of potato chips) claim to contain 2 to 3 servings.

Keep an eye out for fat content too—especially saturated fat. Anything over 3 grams of fat per 100 grams of food can't be labeled as low fat. Anything over 20 grams and warning bells should go off. Health professionals recommend that women like us shouldn't consume more than about 70 grams of fat a day. Remember, fat is packed with calories.

The United States Department of Agriculture recommends a daily intake of about 2,000 calories per day for women and about 2,500 for men. Of course, this will vary depending on your size and how active you are, but it's a good guide. Add up your food diary numbers and you may find you meet this level or even consume less on some days, while on others you eat enough for three of you. But contrary to the ideas behind many of the starvation diets we've all tried, losing weight doesn't mean existing on a few hundred calories a day. Here's a better way to think about it.

Each pound of body fat you carry has an energy content of 3,500 calories. So if you want to lose a pound a week, the amount most experts say is realistic and safe, you'd need to cut your calorie intake by 500 calories a day (500 x 7 days = 3,500). We use this equation: your goal weight x 10 = the number of calories you can eat per day. Take a look at your food diary and see how many calories some of your "guilty pleasures" contain and you'll see that cutting 500 a day is easier than you think. Add a little calorie-burning exercise (see page 73) and you'll be shedding pounds before you can say, "Wow, that was easy."

Buyer Beware

Try not to get too excited if food packaging screams at you from the shelves that it's "low fat," "lite," "less sugar," or one of the many "buy-me-I'll-make-you-thin"-type promises. When something boasts it's 90 percent fat-free, what that means is that it contains 10 percent fat, which is hardly negligible. And remember that "low fat" doesn't mean "low sugar" (i.e., low in calories). If an ice cream bar says it's "reduced sugar," do you know how much sugar was in the original version? If the answer is enough to make your teeth fall out, chances are the reduced version is pretty caloric too. The simple solution to all this confusion is, of course, to reject processed foods as much as possible—definitely steer clear of "diet" foods—and get into the kitchen instead. And before you start protesting that you don't have the time, just think how long it takes to decipher a food label!

Fact

A calorie is basically a unit that measures how much energy your body is able to get from food. Different nutrients in food provide different amounts of calories: for example, fat gives you about 9 calories per gram, alcohol 7, while carbohydrates and protein yield about 4.

Tip

We use this equation: your goal weight x 10 = the number of calories you can eat per day.

Guilty Pleasures

You know they're supposed to be occasional treats that are hardly going to help you lose weight, but somehow you just can't seem to resist them. Here we out some of the biggest offenders when it comes to calorie counts. The good news is you don't have to give these up if you simply cook them the CYT way.

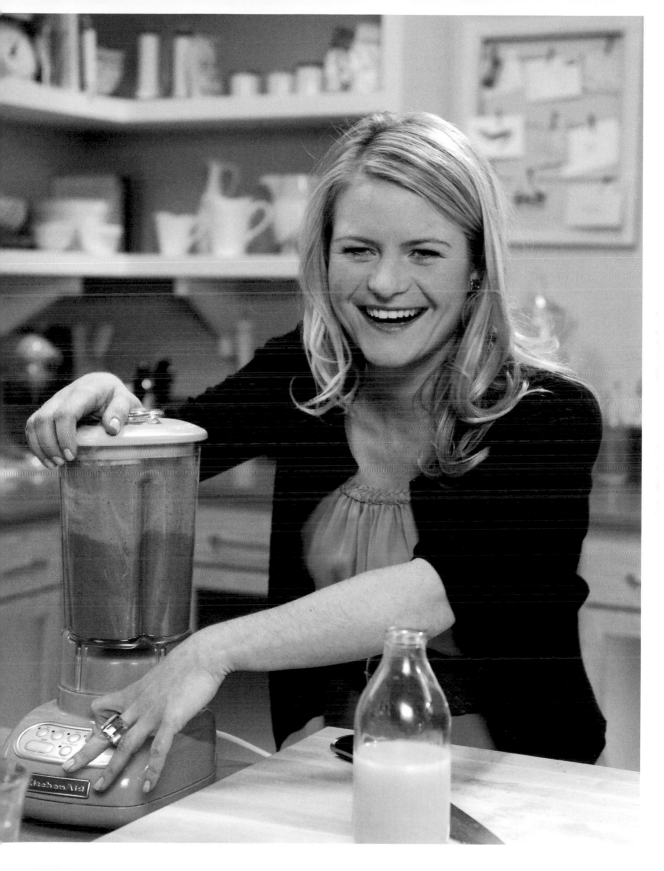

The Surprise Offenders

Generally, we know when we're indulging in a guilty pleasure. As you close your eyes and savor that first bite of rich, luscious, chocolate mousse pie, you know you're not fooling anyone, least of all yourself. It's a decadent thrill that tastes all that much better for being naughty. But what about those everyday foods that look so innocent? The trouble with so-called diet foods is they often taste bland and don't fill you up— leading to the dreaded snack attack later.

Sometimes, despite our most virtuous intentions, the calories just slip past our radar. You think you're munching away on a super-healthy snack when you might just as well have had a buttery scone and be done with it.

Some salty foods contain surprising amounts of sugar. Likewise, products that boast they're "low fat" often compensate by being high in sugar. Don't let foods like these fool you with their healthy façade. It's not that they're outright *bad* for you and that you should give them up—far from it. A fruit smoothie is a great way to get your vitamins, and olive oil has countless beauty and health benefits. Just keep your eye on them—it's worth noting their calorie counts if these items crop up more than two or three times in your food diary.

The Main Offenders

Alcohol—It's fun but full of empty calories, especially if it's dark or sweet.
Cereal—Sugary cereals tend to be higher in calories than high-fiber cereals and far less satisfying.
Granola bars—They may look healthy, but check the label.
Frozen french fries—Watch out for those coated in high-calorie seasoning.
Nuts—They're full of vitamins and minerals, but don't overdo it. Choose raw over roasted.
"Good oils"—They're a dietary essential, just watch how much you slosh on.
Peanut butter—It's good for you, but spread it thin.
Movie popcorn—Smuggle in your own for a fraction of the calories and cost.
Deli sandwiches—Watch out for mayo and other extras.

Store-bought salads—Dressings, croutons, fatty meat, and cheese can turn a light lunch into a calorie-laden pig out.

Fruit smoothies—Go for fruity rather than yogurty and check for added sugar.

Soup and dressings—Check for hidden sugar and cream, or even better make your own (see pages 102, 173, 192).

Toast with butter—It's easy to OD on butter when it melts into the bread.

Veggie burger—Extra fat is often used to boost flavor.

Yogurt—It sounds healthy and often is, but some are high in fat and sugar. Check before you buy.

It's Sugar, but Not as You Know It

Food companies have canny ways of concealing a food's sugar content from us. For instance, they'll list different types of sugars separately. Check the label for:

- Corn syrup
- Dextrose
- Fructose
- Fruit sugar
- Glucose
- High fructose corn syrup/glucose syrup
- Hydrolyzed starch
- Lactose
- Maltose
- Molasses
- Sucrose

A fruit smoothie is a great way to get your vitamins, and olive oil has countless beauty and health benefits.

Calorie Counter
Quick Calorie Guide

The following is a basic guide to the calorie counts of common foods. We're not for one second suggesting you become a calorie bore, but it's here to help you design your own recipe combinations. You don't have to become a slave to calories, but you can take charge of your own waistline.

FRUIT AND VEGETABLES

Apple (1) 50

Apricot (1) 19

   (dried) 1 ounce / 240

Artichoke hearts, half jar 35

Arugula 2 ounces / 10

Asparagus 5 spears (cooked) 33

Banana 90

Beansprouts 2 ounces / 13

Beets 9

Blueberries 5 ounces / 66

Broccoli 3 ounces / 22

Butternut squash 1 ounce / 9

Cabbage 3 ounces / 14

Carrot 1 ounce / 6

Cauliflower 1 ounce / 8

Celery 1 stalk / 3

Cherries 1 ounce / 14

Corn 1 ounce / 31

Corn on the cob 2.5 ounces / 44

Cranberries 1 ounce / 4

Cucumber 1/2 ounce / 1

Dates (1 dried) 54

Eggplant 18

Fennel 1 ounce / 3

Fig 16

   (dried) 32

Grapefruit 68

Grapes 3 ounces / 50

Green beans 1 ounce / 7

Honeydew melon 1 ounce / 8

Kale 1 ounce / 7

Kiwi fruit 25

Leeks 1 ounce / 6

Lettuce 1 ounce / 4

Lychees 1 ounce / 16

Mandarin orange (1 raw) 18

 (canned with juice) 1 ounce / 11

Mango 114

Mushrooms 1 ounce / 3

Nectarine 53

Olives in brine (black) 1 ounce / 51

Olives (green) 1 ounce / 38

Onions 1 ounce / 6

Orange 59

Papaya 1 ounce / 8

Parsnip (cooked) 1 ounce / 18

Peach 1 ounce / 9

Pear 78

Peas 2 1/2 ounces / 51

Peppers 1 ounce / 7

Pickle 5

Pineapple (fresh) 7 ounces / 99

   (canned with syrup) 8 ounces / 158

Plum 32

Potatoes (boiled) 4 ounces / 86

Prunes 2 ounces / 79

Pumpkin 1 ounce / 4

Radish 1 ounce / 3

Raspberries 1 ounce / 7

Rhubarb 1 ounce / 2

Spinach 1 ounce / 7

Scallion 1 ounce / 7

Strawberries 1 ounce / 8

Sweet potato 1 ounce / 24

Tomato 3 ounces / 15

Watermelon 9 ounces / 75

Zucchini 1 ounce / 5

RICE, PASTA, AND GRAINS

Baked beans 14-ounce can / 346

Brown basmati rice 2 ounces / 177

Brown rice 2 1/2 ounces / 267

Couscous 2 ounces / 178

Egg noodles 1 ounce / 109

Jasmine rice 2 ounces / 174

Long grain white rice 2 ounces / 175

Pasta 3 1/2 ounces / 352

Polenta 2 ounces / 232

Popcorn (popped in pan, no butter /
   salt / cheese) 2 1/2 ounces / 282

Rice noodles 1 ounce / 110

Risotto (arborio rice) $2\frac{1}{2}$ ounces / 279
White basmati rice 1 ounce / 200
Whole wheat pasta $3\frac{1}{2}$ ounces / 324

CEREAL AND BREAD PRODUCTS
All Bran $1\frac{1}{2}$ ounces / 112
Bagel $2\frac{1}{2}$ ounces / 215
Baguette 2 ounces / 144
Bran Flakes 1 ounce / 99
Ciabatta $2\frac{1}{2}$ ounces / 174
Chocolate croissant 340
Cornflakes 1 ounce / 112
Croissant (small) 180
English muffin 80
Focaccia 2 ounces / 131
Matzo cracker 34
Medium slice wheat bread 74
Medium slice whole grain bread 83
Medium slice white bread 93
Naan bread 5 ounces / 538
Pita bread $2\frac{1}{2}$ ounces / 199
Oatmeal $1\frac{1}{2}$ ounces / 145
   (not including milk)
Rice cake 27
Rice Krispies 1 ounce / 114
Rye bread 1 ounce / 55
Shredded Wheat (2 pieces) 149
Special K 1 ounce / 112
Table water crackers (1 cracker) 35
Waffle 127
Whole grain bagel 3 ounces / 187

NUTS AND SEEDS
Almonds 1 ounce / 125
Brazil nuts (6 nuts) 137
Cashews 1 ounce / 146
Dry-roasted peanuts 1 ounce / 117
Pine nuts 1 ounce / 195
Pistachios $\frac{1}{2}$ ounce / 92
Pumpkin seeds (1 tablespoon) / 59

DAIRY
Cottage cheese 1 ounce / 29
   (low-fat) 1 ounce / 22
Sour cream $3\frac{1}{2}$ ounces / 362
   (low-fat) $3\frac{1}{2}$ ounces / 181
Goat cheese $\frac{1}{2}$ ounce / 26
Greek yogurt 1 ounce / 36
Hard cheese 1 ounce / 123
Regular yogurt $3\frac{1}{2}$ ounces / 80
   (fat-free) $3\frac{1}{2}$ ounces / 60
Skim milk 7 ounces / 68
1% milk 7 ounces / 98
Cream cheese 1 ounce / 62
Soy milk 7 ounces / 68
Whole milk 7 ounces / 134

MEAT, FISH, EGGS
Bacon (1 slice) 77
Chicken 1 ounce / 42
Chorizo sausage 3 ounces / 250
Cod 1 ounce / 25
Duck 1 ounce / 48
Egg 82
Ham 2 ounces / 57
Lamb (leg) 1 ounce / 58
Lobster 1 ounce / 29
Pork 1 ounce / 42
Roast beef (1 slice) 48
Salami (slice) 18
Salmon $2\frac{1}{2}$ ounces / 149
Scallops $\frac{1}{2}$ ounce / 8
Shrimp 1 ounce / 21
Skate 1 ounce / 18
Steak 1 ounce / 54
Swordfish 1 ounce / 42
Tofu $3\frac{1}{2}$ ounces / 119
Trout 4 ounces / 159
Tuna 5 ounces / 185
   (packed in water) $4\frac{1}{2}$ ounces / 140
   (packed in oil) 5 ounces / 260
Turkey 1 ounce / 33

FATS AND OILS

Butter .2 ounces (a thin spreading) 51
Lard 1 ounce / 249
Low-fat cooking spray (1 spray) 1
Low-fat spread .2 ounces / 25
Margarine .2 ounces / 51
Olive oil 1 tablespoon / 127
Olive-oil spread .3 ounces / 56
Sunflower oil 1 tablespoon / 130
Sesame oil 1 tablespoon / 45

DRINKS

Brandy 1 ounce / 52
Cappuccino 110
   (with skim milk) 60
Champagne 4 ounces / 89
Cola 11 ounces / 135
Fruit juice 3 ounces / 40 to 55
Fruit smoothie 3 ounces / 50
Beer (1 pint) 165
Hot chocolate 330
Latte 260
   (with skim milk) 160
Port 1 1/2 ounces / 79
Red wine 4 ounces / 80
Sherry (dry) 1 1/2 ounces / 58
   (sweet) 1 1/2 ounces / 68
Tomato/vegetable juice 3 1/2 ounces / 20
Vodka 1 ounce / 52
Whiskey 1 ounce / 52
White wine (dry) 4 ounces / 77

CONDIMENTS

Caesar dressing 1 tablespoon / 72
Nutella 1 teaspoon / 68
Chutney 1 teaspoon / 25
Coleslaw 1 ounce / 72
French dressing 1 tablespoon / 71
Honey 1 ounce / 62
Hummus 2 ounces / 150

Jam 1 teaspoon / 25
Ketchup 1 teaspoon / 6
Marmalade 1 teaspoon / 26
Mayonnaise 1 teaspoon / 80
Pesto 1 ounce / 142
Tahini 1 teaspoon / 115
Thousand Island dressing
   1 teaspoon / 19
Tzatziki 1 ounce / 18

SWEET SNACKS

Carrot cake 1 1/2 ounces / 156
Cheesecake 1 ounce / 119
Chocolate bar (milk) 1 ounce / 146
Chocolate cake 1 ounce / 128
Croissant (small) 180
Danish 411
Ice cream (vanilla) 2 1/2 ounces / 145
Jelly doughnut 252
Muffin 161
Regular doughnut 238
Scone 145
Sponge cake with fruit filling
   2 1/2 ounces / 196

APPETIZERS AND SNACKS

Breadstick 20
Potato chips 1 ounce / 148
Garlic bread 2 ounces / 187
Pizza 1 ounce / 66
Quiche Lorraine 1 ounce / 100
Spring roll (vegetable) 2 ounces / 100
Tortilla chips 2 ounces / 240

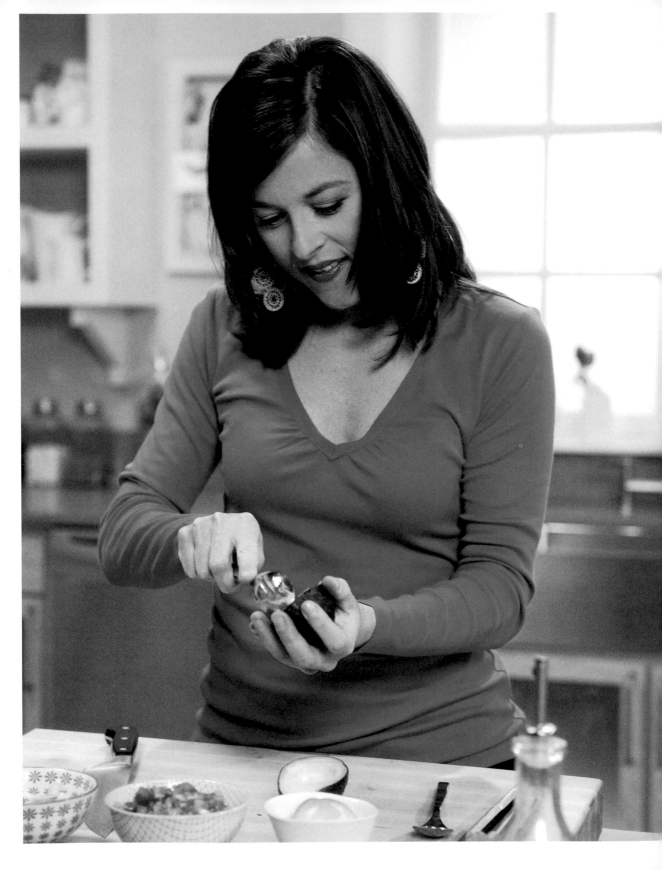

Ingredients for Success

One of the main excuses we hear for cobwebs in the kitchen is lack of time: "I don't get home from work until late and there's no point in cooking." "Takeout is quicker and easier when I'm tired." "There's never any food in the house." "I'm too busy to shop once a week."

Stock up on good things to eat, healthy snacks, and a week's worth of meals. Add a couple of new ingredients each time to experiment with. After all, we all love shopping!

Believe it or not, we can empathize. So many of us nowadays work long hours and fall through the door late in the evening—the last thing any of us want to do is slave over a hot stove (again). And the "nothing in the fridge" excuse—who has the time or energy to shop? Supermarkets can be stressful places.

But if you're serious about putting a dent in your calorie quota, takeout or a frozen meal are not the answers. There are plenty of great-tasting but skinny meals you can make in minutes. The key is having a well-stocked kitchen. One trip to the store, armed with the following list, is all it takes (or even a click of the mouse if you shop online). You don't need to buy it all at once, but these are the sorts of items you'll wonder how you did without.

The following list is made up of cooking basics, condiments, herbs, and spices, all of which form the basis for some really easy, yummy dishes. A well-stocked pantry can be your haven, especially if you consider your freezer as an extension. You already have the basic ingredients for an indulgent Spaghetti Carbonara for example—bacon, pasta, frozen peas, and Parmesan. Why order in?

Some of the meals you can throw together from this list are so basic they don't need recipes. And we hope you'll start to create your own too. We've also included a few of our favorite CYT ingredients to have in the fridge. Obviously, you'll still want to pop into the grocery store from time to time to pick up fresh fruit and vegetables, meat, fish, and dairy products. So we recommend you also grab these goodies each time you go. With your newly stocked cupboards, you'll never use the "nothing to eat" excuse again.

BASICS

Couscous—This is an ultra-quick and easy food. Just pour it over boiling water and let it absorb water.

Eggs—It's the ultimate fast food. Eggs are super filling, and a versatile ingredient.

Garlic—It provides a flavor boost.

Lemons—They're perfect for salad dressing, sauces, sauce ingredients.

Limes

Meringue nests—Just add berries and some fat-free yogurt and you have instant, miniature fat-free desserts.

Rice cakes

Oats—Use it for oatmeal, granola bars, pancakes, or crumble topping.

Onions

Pasta

Popcorn—It's an excellent low-cal snack. Just skip the butter and sprinkle with 2 tablespoons grated cheese.

Pumpkin seeds—They're great in salads. Rumor has it that they're an aphrodisiac too!

Rice (brown, basmati, Thai, and Arborio)

Rice noodles—They're ready in seconds.

Sunflower seeds

HERBS AND SPICES

Basil—Keep a fresh pot on your windowsill if possible.

Bay leaves

Black peppercorns

Cilantro—Get it fresh if possible.

Coriander seeds

Cumin seeds

Dried chili flakes—Should be used sparingly, but it saves having to chop fresh chili peppers.

Fennel seeds

Mint—Use fresh if possible.

Nutmeg

Oregano—Dried is best for a more intense flavor.

Paprika

Parsley—Use fresh and flat-leaf.

Sage—Get it fresh or dried.

Thyme—Dried is fine.

Adding flavor through herbs and spices is an easy route to low-calorie cooking without compromising on taste.

CONDIMENTS

Aged Balsamic vinegar—Makes a fat-free dressing or dip.

Capers

Chicken and beef stock

Cocoa

Cornstarch—Use it for thickening sauces and gravy.

Dried porcini mushrooms

Extra-virgin olive oil—Buy the best

quality you can; the deeper the flavor, the less you'll use.

Fructose—This is a sugar substitute. Use about a fifth less than you would sugar.

Gherkin pickles—They're good as a snack, but they also add flavor when sliced onto a pizza, pasta, or fish.

Honey—It's good for adding sweetness.

Japanese sesame and seaweed seasoning—Sprinkle it over rice and stir-fries for flavor, color, and bite. It makes a good crust for salmon.

Maple syrup

Vegetable bouillon

Miso paste—Just add boiling water for instant miso soup. It's also an easy way to jazz up steamed veggies.

Mustards (Dijon, brown, grainy)— Use it for salad dressings, glazes, and sandwiches.

Olives

Oyster sauce—It is a low-cal, low-fat stir-fry sauce, and is delicious over green veggies or an omelet with scallions.

Panko—These Japanese breadcrumbs are available at the ethnic/ Asian grocery aisle. They're even worth ordering online.

Red wine vinegar

Rice wine vinegar

Sea salt—Experiment by trying Maldon, or one of the many other varieties to enhance flavor.

Soy sauce—Not just for Asian cooking, it also adds depth and color to gravies and sauces. Mix soy, lime, chili flakes, garlic, and coriander for an impressive dip. Or just drizzle it over rice.

Sun-dried tomatoes

Sweet chili sauce—It's perfect for dipping or brushed over shrimp before grilling.

Tabasco sauce—It adds heat to food when you're fresh out of chili peppers or don't want to risk rubbing your eyes after chopping one (ow!).

Tahini—This sesame seed paste is good on rye bread or vegetables and for making hummus.

Thai fish sauce—Okay, it smells *awful*, but trust us, it tastes nothing like that. Once you start using it to add that extra something to dishes, you won't know how you've survived without it.

Vanilla beans—The seeds transform a simple dish like fruit and yogurt into something special.

Wasabi—Because some like it hot!

White wine vinegar

Worcestershire sauce—It creates a flavor explosion in meaty dishes.

FRIDGE AND FREEZER FAVES

Bacon—Believe it or not, a little (regular or turkey) goes a long way.

Bread (pitas, flour tortillas, and whole grain)—Stock them in the freezer.

Cheddar cheese—The stronger the flavor in cheese, the less you'll need to use.

Feta cheese—It's handy for slicing into salads or on pizza.

Dark chocolate—Get at least 70% cocoa solids (if available).

Frozen fruit and vegetables—Buy several, such as peas, lima beans, corn, and summer fruits.

Parmesan—Never buy the grated type! Do it yourself and you'll eat less, especially if you use a microplane grater (see page 52).

Peanut butter—Used sparingly, this is a healthy source of protein. It makes a filling snack on whole grain bread or rice cakes.

Prosciutto

Tofu (solid, not silken)—It's a low-fat protein, great to slice into cubes for last-minute salads and stir-fries.

Half-size bottles of wine or champagne—Buying a whole bottle sometimes means that you have to finish it!

Fat-free yogurt—This is one of the few fat-free versions of a product that really works. You can use this as a substitute for cream, crème fraiche, mayo, or whenever you need something creamy. CYT loves the thick "Greek style."

CANNED FOOD

Anchovies—They're wonderful for adding flavor. Try these (even if you think you don't like them) forked into a paste to add saltiness and depth to dressings, dips, and sauces.

Beans (black, red, white)—They provide a quick, low-fat and easy source of protein to make salads, stews, and Mexican dishes more filling.

Chickpeas—Add them to salads and couscous or toss in the food processor with tahini, garlic, olive oil, lemon juice, and cumin to make hummus.

Salmon—It's handy to flake into salads.

Sardines

Tomatoes—They're a must-have for speedy pasta sauces.

Tuna in water

Kitchen Equipment

Good, fast, fuss-free cooking is all about the equipment you use. You don't have to spend a fortune or clutter your work surfaces with appliances—we're talking about a few choice pieces that will make your food lighter and your life easier. Here are CYT faves.

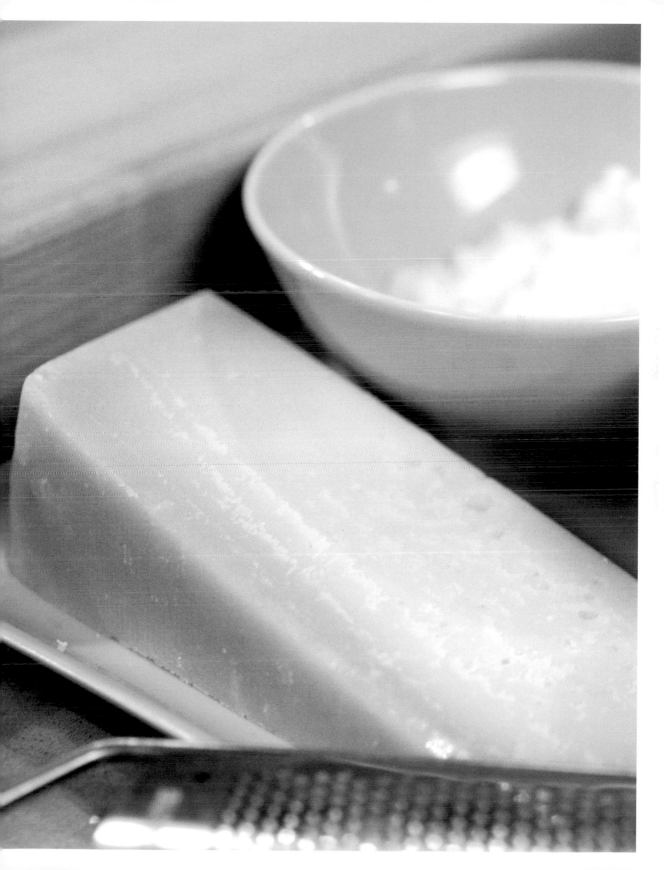

Beautiful plates—What's the point of great-looking food on dull, chipped plates?

Blender—You won't need this and a food processor and a handheld blender unless you're an avid cook (with a big kitchen), but a countertop blender is great if you often make smoothies and soups in large quantities. A glass container is a better investment than plastic. It comes in handy for cocktails, too!

Immersion or stick blender—This is handy for smaller quantities, such as making a soup or smoothie for one or two. It's portable, doesn't take up much room, and is easy to clean.

Hand mixer—Like a handheld blender, this is portable, easy-to-clean, and saves aching arms if you're whisking egg whites or making a cake.

Standing mixer—If you love to bake, you can't live without this workhorse!

Food processor—If you have room, leave this out on your kitchen countertop permanently and you'll use it more often. Once you realize what a time- and labor-saver this is, you'll fall in love. In addition to blending, puréeing and whisking, you'll use it for cakes, making breadcrumbs, and whipping up toppings and spreads.

Ridged griddle or grill pan—For grilling meat, fish, and veggies, this is low- or no-fat fast cooking with an extra smoky flavor. Those barbeque-style griddle marks make you feel like summer is with you all year round.

Paper towels—They're good for blotting grease off food after cooking.

Metal tongs—It's the easiest way to turn food on the grill or in the pan, and to transfer food to plates.

Microplane grater—A kitchen must-have, this makes lightning quick work of citrus zest, ginger, garlic, and cheese. A little goes a long way, so you'll be able to cut down on the amount of cheese you use without noticing.

Good-quality pans—Use two or three saucepans with thick, sturdy bases, tall sides, stay-cool handles, and well-fitting lids. Make sure to have a large, heavy-based, nonstick sauté pan that can be used for searing/flash-frying, and a casserole dish. Stainless steel looks stylish, wears well, and is easy to clean.

Omelet pan—It's perfect for quick meals for one or for toasting nuts. Buy nonstick and you won't need oil.

Pastry brush—It's good for lightly oiling food before cooking.

Pepper grinder

Plastic containers—You'll need airtight ones for storing leftovers or for when you're super-organized and make food in batches to freeze for future meals.

Nonstick roasting pan—Buy one with a sturdy base.

Sharp knives—Even just one super-sharp, high-quality knife is an investment you won't regret.

Spatula—It gets the food to where it needs to be.

Steamer—This is an absolute kitchen essential. Some saucepans come with a steamer that fits on top or you can buy a universal steaming basket that fits into the pan.

Large wok with a lid—If you care for your wok and season it after every use, you'll hardly need any oil. Wok lids are useful when steaming veggies.

Wooden cutting board—It lasts longer than plastic.

Wooden spoons—Perfect for non-stick pans, combining ingredients, and is an all around great tool.

And the Won't-Miss-'Em Items?

If you have any of the following, save space by donating them to a thrift store. Life's too short to use a:

- Blunt knife
- Deep-fat fryer
- Egg poacher
- Electric juicer
- Pasta maker
- Pressure cooker
- Sandwich press
- Yogurt maker

Where Did All the Calories Go?

Now that you've invested in the right equipment, you're ready to get cooking. In addition to choosing lower-calorie foods, what you do with them can make a real difference to your waistline. As you familiarize yourself with the CYT recipes over the following pages, you'll pick up lots of ideas for cooking without the fat or extra calories.

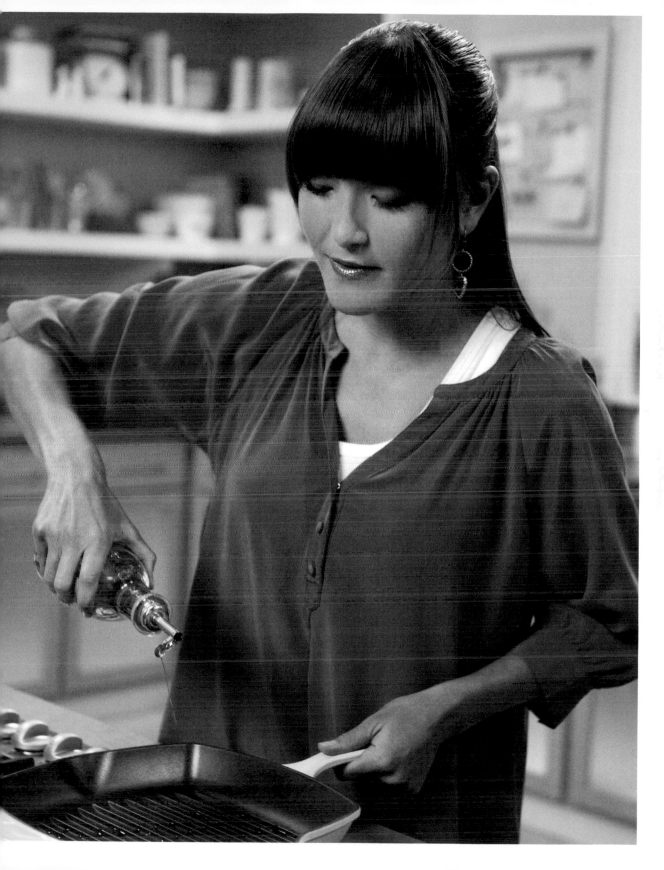

Instead of frying, grill, bake, or stir-fry food using minimal oil in a nonstick pan.

Poaching in a liquid (such as water or stock) is fat-free and an excellent way to keep meat and fish moist and full of flavor. A chicken breast, for example, tastes much more succulent poached in stock than roasted. Just cover the food in liquid, add some herbs or aromatics like carrot, onion, or ginger for a flavor boost. Place a lid on the pan and cook for the same amount of time you would roast, grill, or fry.

Try cutting the amount of sugar in recipes in half (apart from ours, which are already low). It works for most dishes except jam, meringue, and ice cream. Or use one of the sugar substitutes recommended on our list of cupboard ingredients on page 48.

Steaming vegetables preserves more color, flavor, nutrients, and crunch than boiling. You can also use your steamer for fish and meat. If you have a stacking system, such as a bamboo steamer, put the vegetables that will take longest to cook at the bottom.

Buy lean cuts of meat and trim off excess fat before cooking—or ask your butcher to do it for you—and remove the skin from poultry.

Even if a recipe does call for some oil for roasting or frying that doesn't mean all of it has to end up in the dish. You can drain off the fat at any point during cooking and transfer food onto paper towels to blot it before serving.

If you need to prevent sticking, use a pastry brush to put the oil onto the food itself, *not* the pan, griddle, or grill. This way you'll use much less. When you grill meat on a griddle, a common mistake is to add more oil because you think it's stuck. Don't—the meat will release itself from the ridges once it's charred.

When stir-frying in a wok, you only need a tiny drizzle of oil to start. Keep the food moving in the wok and the wok moving over the heat and nothing will stick. Then, to steam the food, add a splash of liquid such as water or soy sauce and put on the wok lid. Most dishes that you think have to be fried are just as successful grilled on a nonstick griddle.

To save on washing up and soul-destroying oven cleaning, line your grill pan and the bottom of your oven with foil to catch drips. You can even line roasting trays with a nonstick sheet.

Comparative Cooking Methods

FILLET OF COD:

Deep fried in batter	445 calories
Pan-fried in 2 teaspoons vegetable oil	150 calories
Grilled	96 calories
Steamed	96 calories

CHICKEN BREAST:

Chicken Kiev from a package	456 calories
Pan-fried in 1 teaspoon butter and 1 teaspoon vegetable oil (no skin)	202 calories
Brushed with 1 teaspoon honey and grilled (no skin)	161 calories
Oven-baked in a foil packet with chicken stock and a dash of white wine	151 calories

Tip

If you need to prevent sticking, use a pastry brush to put the oil onto the food itself, not the pan, griddle, or grill. This way you'll use much less. When you grill meat on a griddle, a common mistake is to add more oil because you think it's stuck. Don't—the meat will release itself from the ridges once it's charred.

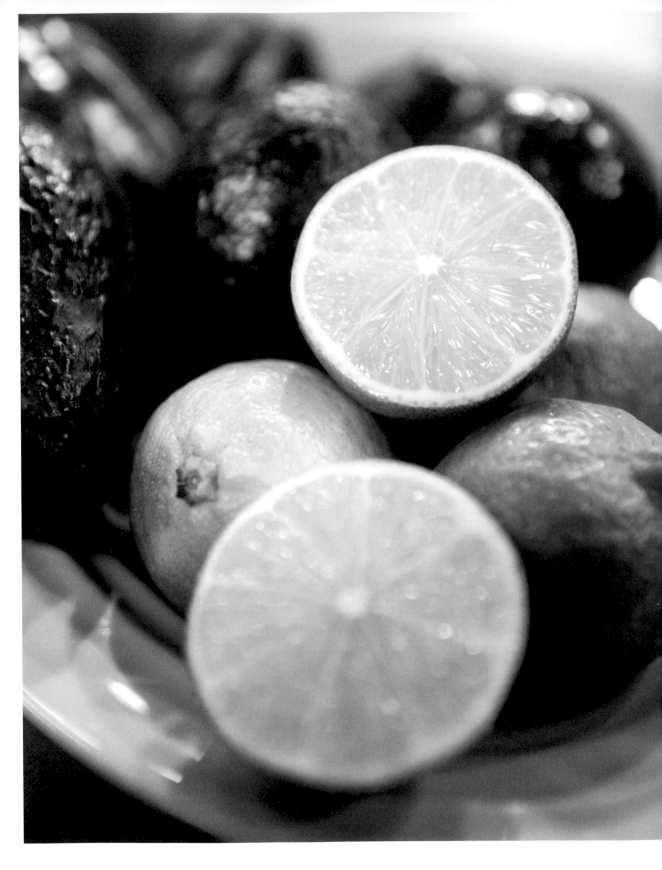

Smart Calorie Swaps

Sometimes you just don't have time to stop and do the math before you indulge. So CYT has done the hard work for you and calculated some simple but brilliant swaps you can make for huge calorie savings without compromising on taste.

Breakfasts

We're all fans of big breakfasts. Believe it or not, if you set yourself up well from the start, it gets your metabolism going so you'll burn more calories during the day. Skip breakfast, on the other hand, and come 11 a.m. you'll be heading out the door on a muffin run, no question. It pays to choose wisely though. The following delicious swaps mean you'll miss out on nothing but calories.

SWAP	FOR
Two thick slices of toast with butter and fruit jam 341 calories	Two medium slices of whole wheat toast with butter and a touch of honey **210 calories**
Croissant with butter and jam 345 calories	Bagel, no butter **289 calories**
Three slices of fried bacon on an English muffin with butter 545 calories	Two slices of grilled bacon with tomato on one slice of wholegrain toast, with no butter **235 calories**
Ham and cheese 3-egg omelet with homefries, toast with butter 890 calories	Slice of Cheese, Vegetable, and Bacon Frittata, page 95 **209 calories**
Cornflakes with whole milk and two teaspoons of sugar 218 calories	Cornflakes with skim milk and half a banana **185 calories**
Eggs Benedict 963 calories	Two slices of smoked salmon and scrambled egg (made with 1% milk and no butter) **220 calories**

Lunches and Snacks

It's very hard to find decent food when you're on the go. Fast-food restaurants, delis, and cafeterias usually rely on fat to add flavor and disguise poor-quality food. Likewise, those convenient snacks you grab aren't so convenient calorie-wise. But we've done the math and worked out a few handy swaps for you.

SWAP **FOR**

Large baked potato with butter and sour cream 770 calories	Healthy Potato Skins, page 115 **420 calories**
Bag of "gourmet" potato chips 240 calories / 50g serving	Two rice cakes with low-fat soft cheese **40 calories**
Extra-mayo tuna sandwiches on white bread 530 calories	Tuna Salad Rolls, page 188 **269 calories**
Cheese platter with bread, butter, cheddar and pickles 700 calories	Tricolor salad with mozzarella, avocado and tomato **500 calories**
Bag of roasted peanuts 300 calories	Large handful of mixed dried fruit **67 calories**
Handful of roasted cashews 155 calories	Handful of mini pretzels **95 calories**

Takeout and Fast Food

If you've simply got to have it (and there's nothing wrong with that), check out the menu before you blurt out your standard order. With a few smart choices, takeout doesn't have to be so terrible (calorie-wise). Better still, cook your own skinny versions with our recipes—so easy they'll be on your plate before the pizza man's knocked on the door.

SWAP **FOR**

Personal pepperoni pizza 2100 calories	Ultimate Personal Sausage and Cheese Pizza, page 137 **475 calories**
Large french fries 610 calories	Sweet Potato Fries, page 99 **89 calories**
Large cheeseburger with bacon 540 calories	Southwestern Turkey Burgers, page 99 **342 calories**
Crispy chicken Caesar salad with dressing and croutons 850 calories	Chicken Caesar Salad, page 107 **469 calories**
Sweet and sour pork with fried rice 513 calories	Sweet and Sour Pork Chops, with Brown Rice, page 168 **465 calories**
Lamb Gyro with yogurt sauce 844 calories	Marinated Lamb Kebabs with Yogurt Sauce, page 184 **315 calories**

Sweet Treats

Pretty soon, your friends will be asking you how you eat so much sugary stuff and still stay slim. Tell them it's our little secret. These sweet cheats are our finest achievement to date.

SWAP **FOR**

Bar of chocolate 260 calories	Chocolate and Cranberry Biscotti, page 217 **76 calories**
Chocolate muffin 630 calories	Banana Chocolate Chip Muffin, page 86 **200 calories**
Slice of strawberry cheesecake 275 calories	One meringue nest with strawberries and fat-free yogurt **105 calories**
Two scoops of ice cream 210 calories	Two scoops of frozen yogurt **150 calories**
Chocolate fudge brownie 580 calories	Chocolate Brownie with Raspberries and White Chocolate Chips, page 208 **291 calories**
Cupcakes 558 calories	Vanilla Cupcakes, page 203 **204 calories**

Drinks

Reducing your calorie intake isn't just about the food you eat. Many soft drinks contain the same number of calories as a decent-sized snack, yet research shows people don't get the same satisfaction from drinks as they do from food. A recent U.S. study found Americans get 22 percent of their daily calories from soft drinks and half the added sugar they consume comes in liquid form. Just cutting back on this one indulgence could add up to serious slimming in no time at all.

SWAP **FOR**

Large latte 265 calories	Small skim-milk latte **120 calories**
Can of Coke 135 calories	Diet Coke **1 calorie**
Mug of hot chocolate with whole milk and marshmallows 360 calories	Mug of cocoa made with skim milk **120 calories**
Large cappuccino with whole milk 155 calories	Regular coffee with skim milk **15 calories**
Pint of carbonated fruit juice 95 calories	Pint of orange juice or lemonade **75 calories**
Glass of pomegranate juice 160 calories	Glass of sparkling water with a squeeze of lime **0 calories**
Mug of tea with whole milk and two sugars 50 calories	Mug of herbal tea **0 calories**
Strawberry milkshake 360 calories	Raspberry, Orange, and Banana Smoothie, page 87 **205 calories**

Alcohol

If you're convinced you never overeat and don't understand why you can't get rid of that last 10 pounds, look at your bar bill. Alcohol is second only to fat in the number of calories it provides, and they're "empty" calories—they won't fuel you or fill you up. There are many health risks associated with alcohol, so the best advice is to consume in moderation, and when you do crave a cocktail, try our tips to save on the calories.

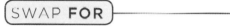

SWAP **FOR**

(all mixers 3 ounces, wine 4 ounces, spirits 1 ounce)

Vodka and cranberry juice 108 calories	Vodka and tomato juice **67 calories**
Pina colada 593 calories	Rum and pineapple juice **102 calories**
Mojito 242 calories	Seabreeze **140 calories**
Bailey's Irish Cream 175 calories	Sambuca **103 calories**
Pint of beer 165 calories	Glass of dry white wine **77 calories**
Mulled wine 227 calories	Glass of red wine **80 calories**
Gin and tonic 120 calories	Gin and diet tonic water **55 calories**
Margarita 145 calories	Glass of champagne **91 calories**

The Skinny Alternatives

There's no need for a rigid plan—one that might work for the duration of the diet, but where does it leave you at the end? More often than not, you're back at square one. The key to *Cook Yourself Thin* is to change your diet, not go on one, and make a few changes to create a lasting difference.

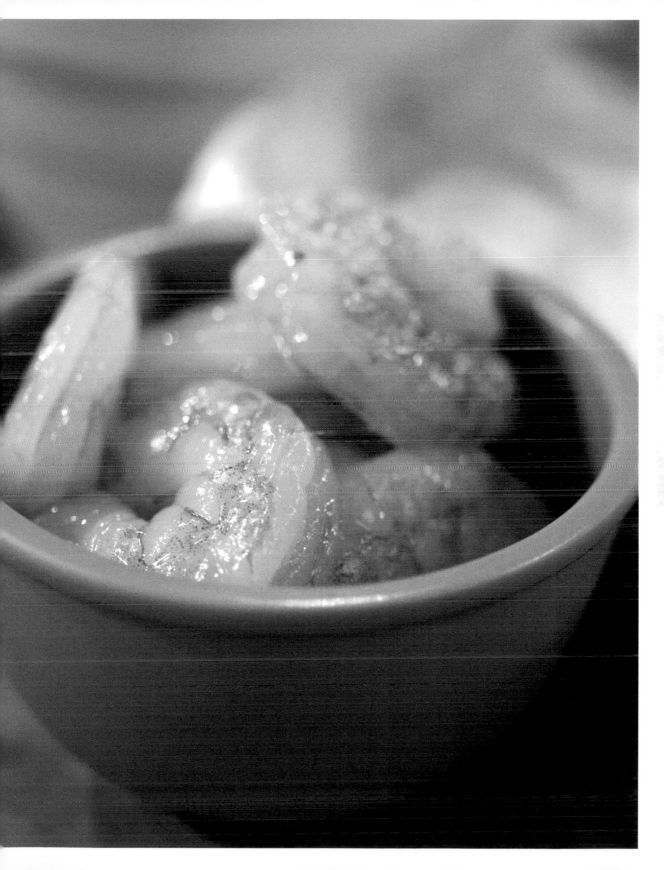

On-the-Run Eater

Blueberry muffin and a large latte from Starbucks	Swap for 2 slices of wholegrain toast (keep bread in the freezer for extra convenience) with butter and jelly and coffee with a splash of milk to **save a whopping 450 calories.**
Early evening fridge raid— two thick slices of white bread and butter That's nearly 400 calories.	Swap for your favorite fruit.
Frozen packaged lasagna and salad and a bottle of beer	Swap for our lasagna, page 110. Make it over the weekend and you can keep it refrigerated for up to three days. **Save an average of 200 calories** compared to supermarket versions.
Swap the beer for—	club soda and you'll **save another 100 calories.**

Sugar Fiend

SWAP **FOR**

Cereal with whole milk	Swap for whole grain cereal, half a banana and skim milk, and you won't need those cookies midmorning.
4 Oreos These really are just an empty sugar hit and 320 calories.	Swap for a piece of fruit. A handful of cherries is 14 calories, and you'll get the same sweet hit.
6 cups of coffee with milk and 2 sugars throughout the day These are adding up 300 extra calories per day.	If you can wean yourself off the sugar, you'll save **240 calories.**
Chicken salad	Watch out for heavy dressings.
Can of orange soda	Swap for a diet version. If you just hate diet soda, then grab an orange and **save over 100 calories.**
Spinach and ricotta ravioli with herby tomato sauce	Good choice
Store-bought chocolate cheesecake 360 calories	Swap for slice of Deep Dark Chocolate Cake, page 197.

Yo-Yo Dieter

SWAP **FOR**

Nothing for Breakfast	This is a bad idea— saving calories first thing usually leads to a need for sugary treats later in the morning
Danish or muffin and a cappuccino mid-morning	Swap for a bowl of oatmeal with skim milk and a regular coffee to **save nearly 300 calories**
Chicken Caesar salad	Swap for our slim version, page 107, and **save over 200 calories.**
After work—3 glasses of white wine, half a plate of fries, and ketchup	Not much food for **nearly 600 calories.** Try alternating a glass of wine with a diet soda or sparkling mineral water and have something to eat before you go out.
Before bed— cheese and crackers Another 540 calories.	If you know you're going to get home hungry, keep some 5-minute meals on hand, like miso soup with noodles, or heat up some soup you made over the weekend.

Comfort Food Craver

SWAP **FOR**

BLT with mayo and creamy tomato soup	Swap for our Turkey BLT and Tomato Fennel Soup, page 173
Five shortbread cookies These very quickly add up to 335 calories.	A small bowl of popcorn (no butter or cheese) is only **60 calories**—the perfect comfort snack.
Macaroni and cheese can easily contain over 800 calories... gulp!	See ours, page 167 **(517 calories).**

Exercise

We're not suggesting you have to exercise—merely that you might like to from time to time as a smart way to earn yourself an extra calorie allowance. You might even be doing it without noticing—your walk to work, busting moves on the dance floor, a night of passion. It all adds up.

Exercise will help speed weight loss and is essential to maintaining a healthy lifestyle. So next time you've overindulged, you can restore the balance in no time at all. Here is a list of activities to help get you started.

Calories Used in Common Physical Activities
(for a 154-pound Person)

ACTIVITY	30 MINUTES	1 HOUR
Aerobics	240 calories	480 calories
Basketball (vigorous)	220 calories	440 calories
Bicycling (less than 10 mph)	145 calories	290 calories
Bicycling (greater than 10 mph)	295 calories	590 calories
Dancing	165 calories	330 calories
Golf (walking and carrying clubs)	165 calories	330 calories
Heavy yard work (chopping wood)	220 calories	440 calories
Hiking	185 calories	370 calories
Light gardening / yard work	165 calories	330 calories
Running / jogging (5 mph)	295 calories	590 calories
Stretching	90 calories	180 calories
Swimming (slow freestyle laps)	255 calories	510 calories
Walking (3.5 mph)	140 calories	280 calories
Walking (4.5 mph)	230 calories	460 calories
Weight lifting (general light workout)	110 calories	220 calories
Weight lifting (vigorous effort)	220 calories	440 calories

Source: Adapted from http://www.cdc.gov/healthyweight/physical_activity/index.html

Recipes

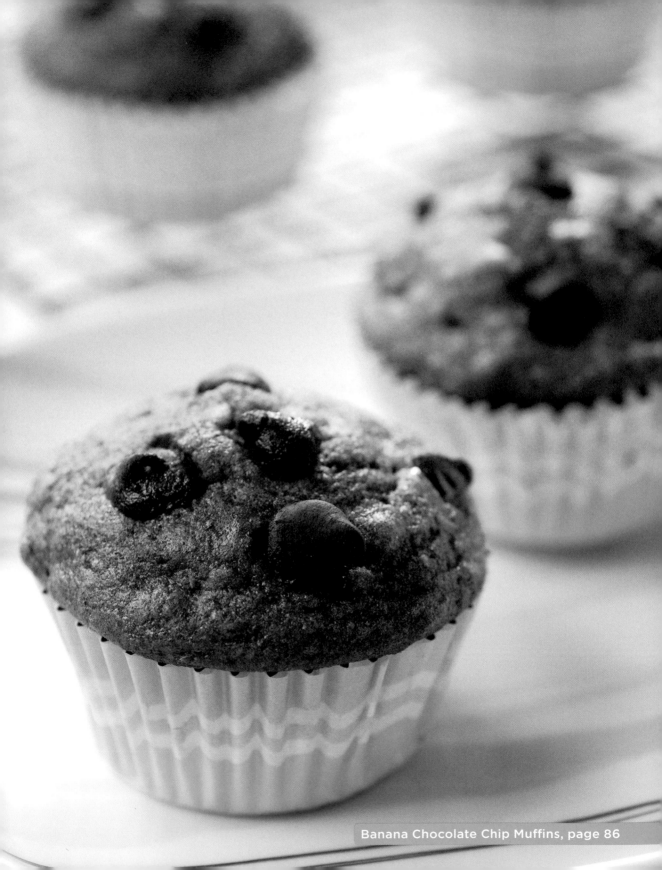

Banana Chocolate Chip Muffins, page 86

Breakfast

The Better for You Breakfast Sandwich

A few savvy choices give you all the flavor and satisfaction of that greasy bacon, egg, and cheese sandwich with just a fraction of the fat and almost none of the guilt. Save even more calories by skipping half the bread.

SERVES 4
Calories per serving: 306

2	tablespoons white vinegar
4	whole wheat English muffins
4	slices of low-fat cheese
4	deli-thin slices low-sodium ham
4	large eggs
4	slices tomato
	Spritz of olive oil
½	tablespoon dried oregano
	Salt, to taste
	Pepper, to taste

1. PREHEAT the oven to 350 degrees. Fill a large, deep skillet of water to a depth of 4 inches. Add vinegar and bring to a steady simmer.

2. ARRANGE the muffin halves on a baking sheet and using a round biscuit cutter, cut each slice into a round. Cut the cheese slices into 3-inch rounds using a round biscuit cutter. Place a slice of cheese on each of the bottom halves. Cut the slice of ham into shreds or ribbons and place on top of the cheese. Transfer to the oven and bake until cheese melts and top halves are toasted, about 4 minutes.

3. MEANWHILE, cut 4 slices from the tomato and spritz each slice with some olive oil. In a separate nonstick sauté pan over medium-high heat, sauté the tomato slices for 1 minute on each side. Then season with salt, pepper, and dried oregano. Set aside.

4. BREAK one egg into a small bowl. Hold the edge of the bowl close to the simmering water and gently tilt the bowl to pour the egg into the water. Repeat with the remaining three eggs. Cook until whites are solid and the yolk is still runny, about 3 minutes. Carefully remove the eggs one at a time with a slotted spoon. Transfer to a plate with paper towels to drain.

5. REMOVE the toasted muffin halves with cheese and ham from the oven and transfer to a plate. Place a slice of sautéed tomato on top of the ribbons of ham and top with a poached egg. Season with salt and pepper and top with the other half of each muffin. Serve immediately.

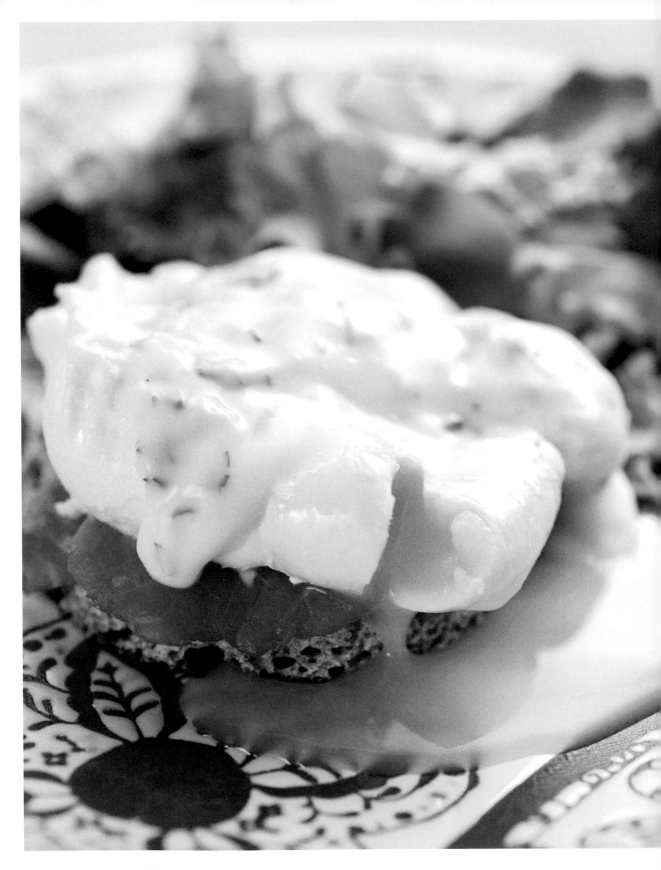

Eggs Benedict on a Muffin with Garlic Aïoli

This brunch staple gets a slimming makeover when we replace that fatty Canadian bacon with a few slices of smoked salmon. Garlic and a little lemon transform low-fat mayo into an aioli worth getting out of bed for.

SERVES 4
Calories per serving, eggs Benedict on a muffin: 178
Calories per serving, garlic aïoli: 145

For the eggs:
8   fresh chives
     Salt, to taste
     Pepper, to taste
2   tablespoons white vinegar
4   large eggs
2   whole wheat English muffins
8   slices smoked salmon (4 ounces)
1   cup mixed baby greens

For the garlic aïoli:
1 ½ cups reduced fat mayonnaise
2   cloves garlic, coarsely chopped
2   tablespoons fresh lemon juice
1   teaspoon finely chopped
     lemon zest
     Salt, to taste
     Freshly ground pepper, to taste
2   tablespoons water, warm
2   tablespoons finely chopped, fresh,
     flat-leaf parsley

1. TRIM 1 ½ inches from the tops of the chives, and reserve for garnish. Finely chop remaining chives, and transfer to a small bowl. Set aside.

2. FILL a large, deep skillet of water to a depth of 4 inches. Add vinegar and bring to a steady simmer. Break an egg into a small bowl, hold the edge of the bowl close to the water, and tilt the egg into the water. Repeat with the remaining eggs. Cook until whites are cooked through, but yolk is still runny, about 3 minutes. Carefully remove the eggs, one at a time, with a slotted spoon, and drain on paper towels.

3. TOAST the English muffin halves, and cut into 3-inch rounds using a biscuit or cookie cutter. Place a poached egg on the cut side of each muffin, and drape a slice of smoked salmon on each egg. Divide the greens among the muffins and mound over the smoked salmon. Spoon the sauce over and around the eggs Benedict, garnish with remaining chives, and serve.

> **Tip**
> Low-fat buttermilk has a creamy texture and richness from the acidity that can substitute for higher-fat dairy products such as cream and sour cream.

Sweet 'N' Spicy Breakfast Hash with Tofu

We jettisoned the belly-busting corned beef and went with tasty baked tofu, hooking it up with some nice spice notes when it mingles with jalapeño, red onion, and a little hot sauce. Drop a poached egg on top and it's breakfast done right.

SERVES 4
Calories per serving: 322

For the hash:

1	tablespoon vegetable oil
1	cup finely chopped red onion
1	large jalapeño, chopped
	Kosher salt, to taste
	Freshly ground pepper
4	cups peeled, roasted sweet potatoes, 1-inch cubed
2	tablespoons ketchup
4	tablespoons Worcestershire sauce
8	ounces baked tofu, diced
4	teaspoons chopped parsley

For serving:

scallions, chopped
Hot sauce
Ketchup

1. IN A NONSTICK SKILLET, heat the oil over medium-high heat. Add the onions and the jalapeño and season with salt and pepper. Cook until golden, about 5 minutes.

2. ADD the cubed potatoes, ketchup, and Worcestershire sauce and season with salt. Press the mixture down into the skillet, reduce the heat to medium, and cook until golden, about five to seven minutes.

3. WHILE THE POTATOES ARE COOKING, cut the tofu into quarter-inch dice, about the same size as the potatoes. When potatoes are cooked, gently add diced tofu.

4. PLACE the hash on a plate and top with parsley. Serve with scallions, hot sauce, and ketchup, if desired.

Stuffed French Toast Sundaes

Here's a breakfast question for you: What's not to like about low-cal, low-fat baked wheat bread French toast topped with creamy ricotta, dark berries, and rich maple syrup? So it's a loaded question, but to us it's the best reason to rise and shine we've heard in a long time. It's a sundae to start your Sunday!

SERVES 2
Calories per serving: 353

1   whole egg
1   egg white
2   tablespoons skim milk
½   teaspoon ground cinnamon
1   teaspoon honey
4   slices whole wheat bread, crusts removed
½   cup part-skim ricotta cheese
¼   cup raspberries
½   cup blackberries
2   tablespoons pure maple syrup

1. PREHEAT the oven to 375 degrees.

2. IN A BOWL, whisk together the egg, egg white, milk, cinnamon, and honey. Spray a nonstick muffin pan with calorie-free vegetable spray. Carefully dip each slice of the bread into the egg/milk mixture and press it into the muffin pan. Bake at 375 degrees for 12 minutes until crisp.

3. MEANWHILE, in a small bowl, mix together the ricotta cheese until smooth. Spoon equal amounts of the ricotta mixture into each of the bread cups and top with berries. Drizzle the maple syrup on top.

Portobello Mushroom Benedict with Roasted Red Pepper Sauce

You'll never go back to muffins again after you experience eggs Benedict with the elegant addition of portobellos. And roasted red pepper sauce only tastes decadent as a full-flavor, low-fat stand-in for the usual scale-tipping hollandaise.

SERVES 4
Calories per serving, portobello Benedict: 183
Calories per serving, roasted red pepper sauce: 70

For the portobello Benedict:
4   portobello mushrooms,
    gills removed
1   tablespoon olive oil
1   garlic clove
2   10-ounce bags of baby spinach
1   teaspoon fresh lemon juice
1   teaspoon lemon zest
    Pinch nutmeg
1/2 teaspoon salt
1/4 teaspoon freshly ground pepper
4   tablespoons Parmesan cheese

For the roasted red pepper sauce (serves 8):
1   4-ounce jar roasted red peppers,
    drained and finely chopped
3/4 cup reduced fat mayonnaise
1   ounce capers, drained
1   tablespoon parsley, chopped

1. FOR THE PORTOBELLO BENEDICT: Preheat the oven to 425 degrees. Lightly oil a baking sheet.

2. USING AN ORDINARY SPOON, remove the gills from each mushroom cap and place the caps on the oiled baking sheet. Bake the mushrooms for 10 to 12 minutes or until tender. Remove from the oven and set aside.

3. IN A SMALL SAUTÉ PAN over medium heat, add the olive oil, garlic, and spinach. Cook for 3 to 5 minutes, tossing occasionally until wilted. Add the lemon juice, lemon zest and nutmeg.

4. IN A BLENDER or small food processor combine the sauce ingredients and pulse until creamy.

5. USING A SPOON, evenly distribute the spinach onto the 4 portobello caps. Top each one with a poached egg, some roasted red pepper sauce, and some grated Parmesan cheese. Serve.

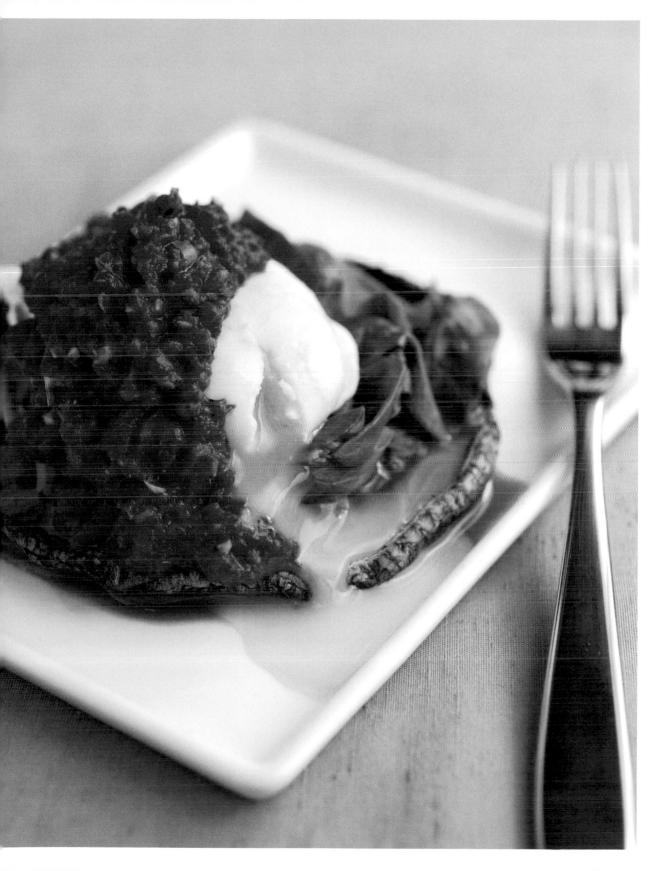

Banana Chocolate Chip Muffins

A little chocolate goes a long way in these hearty muffins powered by wheat flour and heart-healthy oat bran. And tangy low-fat buttermilk takes the place of heavy cream without making a fuss about it.

MAKES 12 MUFFINS
Calories per serving: 200

1	cup all-purpose flour
1	cup whole wheat flour
1/2	cup rolled oats
2	teaspoons ground cinnamon
2	teaspoons baking powder
1	teaspoon baking soda
1/2	teaspoon salt
1	ripe banana, mashed
1/4	cup chopped walnuts
1/2	cup light brown sugar
2	tablespoons vegetable oil
2	large organic eggs
1 1/4	cups reduced-fat buttermilk
1	teaspoon pure vanilla extract
2	tablespoons chocolate chips

1. PREHEAT the oven to 400 degrees. Line a 12-muffin tray with paper liners. Set aside.

2. IN A STANDING MIXER, combine the all-purpose flour, wheat flour, rolled oats, ground cinnamon, baking powder, baking soda, salt, and mashed banana and blend on low speed for 2 minutes. Add the walnuts, brown sugar, vegetable oil, eggs, and reduced-fat buttermilk and blend for 2 minutes on medium speed. Add the vanilla extract and mix until well combined.

3. USING an ice cream scoop, portion the batter evenly into the muffin tin and top each muffin with 3 to 4 chocolate chips. Bake at 400 degrees for 15 minutes. Once they are baked through, remove them from the oven and let cool. Serve.

Tip

Keep your muffins fresher longer: store them in a plastic bag or an airtight container.

Raspberry, Orange, and Banana Smoothie

Take bananas, juice and raspberries for a spin in the blender and come away with a thick, rich, and totally satisfying drink that's an ideal mid-morning appetite slayer.

This is ideal as a mid-morning drink to boost your energy levels.

SERVES 2
Calories per serving: 205

1   cup fresh raspberries
½   cup chopped banana
2½ cups freshly squeezed orange juice

1. PLACE the ingredients into the bowl of a blender and whip up until smooth.

Tips

1. You could take this smoothie to work for a great breakfast or snack in an empty bottle or jar. Just shake before drinking.

2. This smoothie can be stored in the refrigerator for up to 24 hours.

Lemon and Poppyseed Muffins

A little bit sweet but also sporting the savory tang of buttermilk, these versatile muffins fit in just about anywhere. Serve them as dessert, breakfast, or in place of coffee cake as part of a mid-morning snack.

MAKES 12 MUFFINS
Calories per serving: 200

1½ cups white rice flour
1½ cups finely ground almonds
2   teaspoons baking powder
1   teaspoon baking soda
¼   teaspoon salt
1   tablespoon poppy seeds
     zest of 1 large lemon
2   cups peeled and finely grated zucchini
3   large eggs
½   cup of buttermilk
¾   cup sugar
2   teaspoons lemon extract

1. PREHEAT the oven to 350 degrees. Line a 12-muffin tray with paper liners.

2. COMBINE the dry ingredients (flour, almonds, baking powder, baking soda, salt, poppy seeds) and set aside.

3. IN A SMALL BOWL, combine the lemon zest and the zucchini.

4. BEAT the eggs and sugar with a handheld or standing mixer for 3 minutes, until pale and creamy.

 Tip

The key to successful muffins lies in not overworking or overbeating the mixture. Use the spatula and work really fast once the eggs and the sugar have gotten their "air and stability workout" with the electric beaters.

5. **ADD** the zucchini, buttermilk, lemon zest, and lemon extract and beat again. Using a spatula, beat in the dry ingredients until they are all mixed in, working quickly.

6. **SPOON** even amounts of the batter into each muffin liner. Bake for 30 minutes. Remove from oven, let cool, and serve.

> **Tip**
>
> Fill the muffins right up to the top. There should be just the right amount of mixture for muffin cases. It's nice to have a good muffin top: generous and fluffy and cracked is wonderful.

Homemade Granola

Granola seems like a healthy way to start your day, but with all the fat and calories lurking in store-bought varieties, you may as well eat a box of donuts. When you make it yourself, you get back to the healthy, nutty ideal that gave granola its great reputation and taste in the first place.

MAKES 15 BREAKFASTS
Calories per serving: 270

5	cups jumbo rolled oats
1	cup slivered almonds
1	cup sunflower seeds
1	teaspoon cinnamon
1/4	teaspoon salt
1/4	cup runny honey, change to 1 cup honey, if too dry
1/4	cup dried cherries
1/4	cup dried cranberries
1	cup barley flakes/rye flakes (optional)
1/2	cup flaxseed (optional)

1. PREHEAT the oven to 350 degrees. Line a baking sheet with parchment paper cut to size.

2. PLACE the oats, almonds, sunflower seeds, and salt onto the baking sheet and place in the oven at 350 degrees for 10 minutes to heat it up.

3. DIP dip your measuring cup into hot water, discard water, and measure the honey. Run the warm honey over the hot granola and give a good stir to coat evenly.

4. RETURN pan to the oven for the final 30 minutes. Toss the ingredients halfway through their cooking time in order to cook evenly.

5. REMOVE from the oven and add the dried berries, flaxseed, cinnamon, and the barley or rye flakes (if using). Cool well before storing or it will lose its crunch.

6. STORE in an airtight container. Serve with yogurt and fruit for breakfast, or with milk.

> *Tip*
>
> By all means, replace the dried berries with dried pineapple, papaya, or mango, and the almonds with dried coconut for a tropical twist. In this instance, replace the cinnamon with $1/2$ teaspoon ground ginger.

Omelets with Roasted Tomatoes

Lighten up your morning with an omelet sporting more whites than yolks, and fill it with your choice of low-fat savory fillings. Earthy goat cheese and spinach, a Western classic with peppers and ham, sharp cheddar and scallion, or the intensified flavor of sweet, roasted tomatoes all turn a plain omelet into a revelation.

SERVES 4
Calories per serving, omelet: 137
Calories per serving, spinach goat cheese filling: 109
Calories per serving, Western filling: 145
Calories per serving, cheddar scallion filling: 60
Calories per serving, roasted tomatoes: 49

4   whole eggs plus 8 egg whites
$\frac{1}{2}$ teaspoon salt
$\frac{1}{4}$ teaspoon pepper
4   teaspoons un-salted butter

1. BEAT 4 whole eggs and 8 egg whites, with $\frac{1}{4}$ teaspoon salt and $\frac{1}{8}$ teaspoon pepper with a fork until blended.

2. HEAT 2 teaspoons of the butter in a 10-inch nonstick skillet over medium-high heat. When the butter begins to turn a golden brown color, pour in the eggs, and stir with a wooden spoon as if you were making scrambled eggs, shaking the pan as you stir, until the eggs thicken, 5 to 10 seconds.

3. SPRINKLE one of the fillings, if desired, over the center third of the omelet. Use a spatula to fold the back third of the omelet over the center, and then fold the front third over. Turn the omelet out onto a plate and serve with roasted tomatoes (below).

SPINACH-GOAT CHEESE FILLING

    9-ounce package baby spinach
$\frac{1}{2}$ teaspoon salt
3   ounces goat cheese, crumbled

4. **COMBINE** about half of the spinach, and the salt, in the nonstick skillet and cook, covered, over medium-low heat until wilted, 1 to 2 minutes. As spinach wilts, you'll have room to add the rest of the spinach. Continue cooking until wilted, 3 to 4 minutes total.

5. **DIVIDE** the spinach and cheese evenly between each omelet before folding.

WESTERN FILLING

2   teaspoons olive oil
1   red or green bell pepper (or $\frac{1}{2}$ each)
$\frac{1}{4}$ red onion, chopped (about $\frac{1}{2}$ cup)
$\frac{1}{4}$ teaspoon salt
4   ounces ham, chopped (could cut ham to 2 ounces)
3   ounces pepper-jack cheese, grated

6. **HEAT** the oil in the nonstick skillet over medium heat. Add the pepper, onion, and salt, cover, and cook until vegetables are lightly browned and softened, about 5 minutes. Remove from heat.

7. **DIVIDE** the vegetable mixture, ham and cheese evenly between each omelet before folding.

CHEDDAR-SCALLION FILLING

2   ounces ($\frac{1}{2}$ cup) shredded sharp cheddar cheese
2   scallions, trimmed and chopped

8. **SPRINKLE** half of the cheese and half of the scallions over each omelet before folding.

ROASTED TOMATOES
SERVES 4

Nonstick cooking spray
6   large roma tomatoes, stem ends trimmed,
    halved lengthwise (about 1 1/2 pounds)
1/2   teaspoon salt
1/4   teaspoon pepper
1/2   teaspoon dried thyme
1   tablespoon olive oil

9. ARRANGE the rack in the upper third of the oven and preheat oven to 450 degrees. Spray a baking sheet with nonstick cooking spray.

10. ARRANGE tomatoes, cut sides up, in one layer in the pan and sprinkle with salt, pepper, and thyme. Drizzle with the oil. Roast until tomatoes shrivel and begin to brown on the edges, 35 to 40 minutes. Serve warm or at room temperature.

Cheese, Vegetable, and Bacon Frittata

Eggs get the European treatment in this fluffy frittata, seasoned with a medley of chopped fresh herbs. The key is olive oil spray for the gently sautéed veggies, while crumbled bacon and grated Romano turn it into a tempting brunch main course you'll find yourself serving again and again.

SERVES 6
Calories per serving: 209

6   large eggs
¼   cup 1% milk
¼   pound bacon, cooked and rough chopped
¼   cup grated Romano cheese
    Olive oil spray
1   garlic clove, chopped
¼   cup white onion, diced
½   cup asparagus, sliced into ½ inch sticks
1   large zucchini, sliced into half moons
½   cup assorted mushrooms, sliced thinly
¼   cup tomato, chopped
1   tablespoon fresh basil, chopped
1   tablespoon fresh oregano, chopped
1   tablespoon fresh thyme, chopped

1. TURN broiler on to low setting. In a medium bowl, whisk eggs, milk, bacon, and ¼ cup grated Romano. Set aside.

2. HEAT a medium nonstick sauté pan over medium-high heat. Spray with olive oil. Add the minced garlic and chopped onion and cook for 2 minutes.

3. ADD asparagus and zucchini to pan. Sauté 4 to 5 minutes.

4. ADD mushrooms, chopped tomatoes, and freshly chopped basil, oregano, and thyme and sauté for another 2 minutes. Add the egg mixture and cook for 4 to 5 minutes until the bottom has set and browned.

5. PLACE the frittata into the oven and broil until golden and fluffy. Remove from pan and cut into 6 portions.

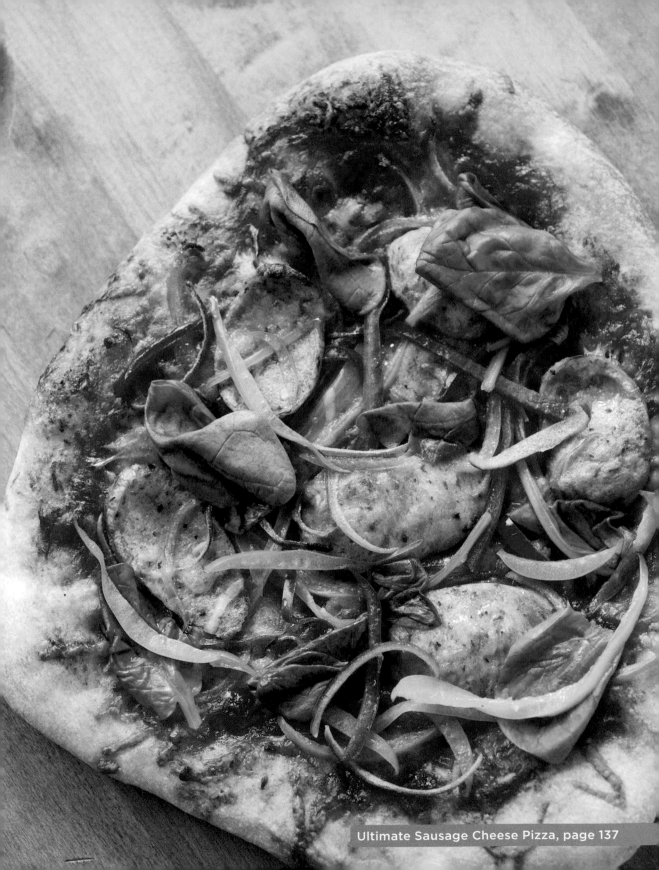

Ultimate Sausage Cheese Pizza, page 137

Mains

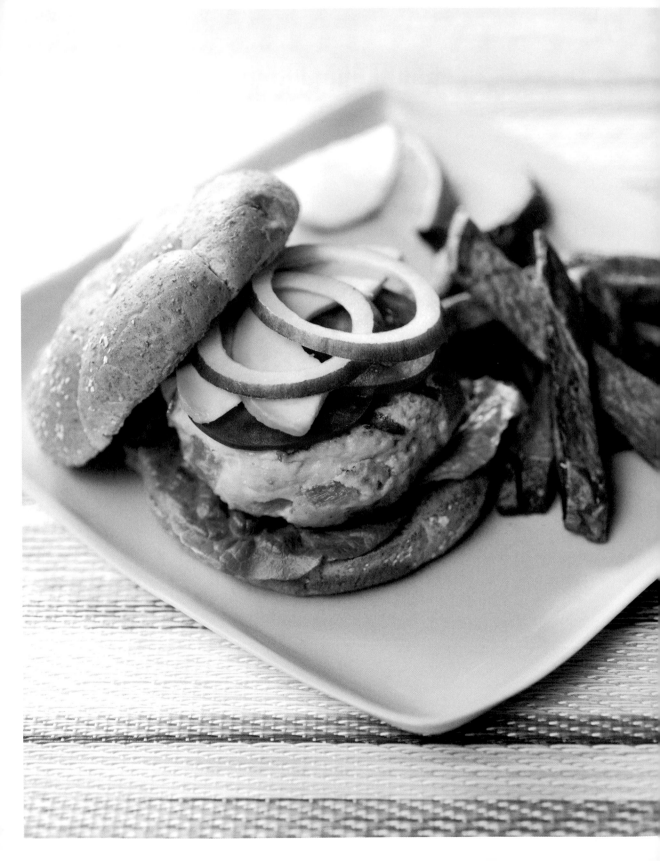

Southwestern Turkey Burgers with Sweet Potato Fries

Let the flavors of the Southwest transport you with burgers so full of flavor and fun you'll need a pinch to remind yourself you aren't scrapping your diet. The avocado slices replace the usual mayo and add richness and flavor. Topped off with baked sweet potato fries, this festive spa food feels positively indulgent.

SERVES 4
Calories per serving, turkey burger: 342
Calories per serving, sweet potato fries: 89

Sweet Potato Fries
2   sweet potatoes
1   tablespoon olive oil
½   teaspoon chili powder
½   teaspoon garlic powder
¼   teaspoon salt, plus more
     for sprinkling
     Juice of ½ lime

Turkey Burger
1⅓ pounds lean ground turkey
     4-ounce can diced green chiles,
     drained
¼   teaspoon salt
¼   teaspoon black pepper
2   3 spritzes canola oil in a mister

3   ounces 50%-reduced-fat
     pepper-jack cheese,
     cut into 8 thin slices
4   whole wheat kaiser rolls
     Romaine lettuce leaves
     Tomato, sliced
     Red onion, sliced
½   avocado, sliced

1. FOR THE SWEET POTATO FRIES, preheat the oven to 425 degrees.

2. WASH and dry the potatoes and, with the skin on, slice into ½-inch thick rounds; cut the rounds into ½-inch thick finger-shaped pieces. Toss the potatoes in a bowl with the oil, chili powder, garlic powder, and salt.

3. ON A BAKING SHEET, spread the potato fries in a single layer and roast, stirring every 10 minutes, until brown and tender, 30 to 35 minutes. Remove from the oven, transfer to a platter or bowl and sprinkle with a little more salt.

4. MEANWHILE IN A LARGE BOWL, mix the lean ground turkey with the diced chiles and season with salt and pepper. Shape into patties and refrigerate until ready to cook.

5. HEAT a large grill pan or nonstick skillet on medium heat and spritz with canola oil. Add the turkey patties to the grill pan and cook until browned on one side, about 4 minutes. Flip, reduce the heat to low, cover (if using a skillet), and cook until the juices run pale pink, about 4 more minutes. Top with the reduced-fat pepper-jack cheese during the last minute.

6. TOAST the rolls in the oven or in a toaster oven. Alternatively, grill them 1 minute on each side.

7. TO ASSEMBLE: On a platter, place the fries and a burger on a bun and top with lettuce, tomato, onion, and avocado slices. Squeeze lime juice over the fries and serve.

Tip

Adding chopped vegetables, like the diced green chilies in this recipe, to lean ground turkey keeps the meat juicy and boosts flavor.

Penne alla "Not-ka"

We love that this pasta dish is so easy to make and satisfying, yet has a fraction of the fat and calories you'd expect. Paired with a small salad, it's the perfect weeknight meal.

SERVES 4
Calories per serving: 371

2	teaspoons olive oil, plus extra for serving
3	cloves garlic
$\frac{1}{2}$	cup chopped red onion
$\frac{3}{4}$	teaspoon salt
1	14-ounce can diced tomatoes or whole tomatoes in juice, pureed in a food processor
	Pinch red pepper flakes
8	ounces penne
$\frac{1}{4}$	cup whipping cream
6	tablespoons evaporated nonfat milk
$\frac{1}{3}$	cup grated Parmesan cheese
$\frac{1}{4}$	cup shredded fresh basil
$\frac{1}{8}$	teaspoon black pepper

1. BRING a large pot of salted water to a boil for the penne.

2. IN A LARGE SAUCEPAN, heat the 2 teaspoons oil with the garlic over low heat until the garlic begins to brown, about 3 minutes. Add the onion and $\frac{1}{4}$ teaspoon salt, cover, and cook until the onion is softened, about 2 more minutes. Add the tomato, $\frac{1}{2}$ teaspoon salt, and the red pepper flakes. Bring to a simmer, reduce the heat and simmer very gently 10 minutes. Stir in the cream and evaporated milk and simmer 1 more minute.

3. MEANWHILE, after the sauce has cooked 5 minutes, add the penne to the boiling water and cook until just shy of al dente, about 6 minutes. Drain, reserving about $\frac{1}{2}$ cup pasta water. Add the drained penne to the saucepan and simmer until the penne is al dente, 1 to 2 minutes, adding a little of the pasta cooking water if the mixture is dry. Stir in $\frac{1}{4}$ cup of the Parmesan, the basil, and black pepper.

4. TO SERVE, divide pasta between 4 serving bowls. Drizzle each serving with $\frac{1}{2}$ teaspoon olive oil, and sprinkle with the remaining Parmesan.

French Onion Soup

We slim down this classic French starter by using just a sliver of nutty Gruyere and don't even miss the extra cheese. Same gooey melt, same transporting aroma, same warm comfort food.

SERVES 4
Calories per serving: 302

- ¼ cup olive oil
- 2 large white onions, halved lengthwise and cut into ¼-inch-thick slices crosswise
- 4 sprigs fresh thyme
- 2 bay leaves
- ¼ teaspoon salt
- ¼ teaspoon freshly ground pepper
- ⅓ cup dry white wine
- 4 cups low-sodium chicken stock
- 4 (1-inch-thick) slices whole wheat baguette, toasted and cooled
- 2 ounces Gruyere, shaved into paper-thin slices with a cheese plane or vegetable peeler

1. PREHEAT the oven to 400 degrees.

2. HEAT the oil in a large saucepan over medium heat. Add the onions, thyme, bay leaves, salt, and pepper and cook, stirring occasionally, until the onions are golden (not brown) and nearly melting, about 45 minutes. Stir in wine and simmer, stirring occasionally, until reduced by half. Stir in stock and simmer, stirring occasionally, for 15 minutes.

3. PLACE 4 soup crocks or ovenproof bowls (no larger than 4 inches round) on a rimmed baking sheet. Place a baguette slice in each crock. Divide the soup among the bowls and top each with a single layer of cheese slices.

4. TRANSFER to the oven and bake until cheese melts and is golden brown in spots and soup is bubbling, about 10 minutes. Serve immediately.

The high-calorie element of French onion soup is the traditional thick cap of Gruyere cheese. In this version, a very thin slice of Gruyere is melted on top of the soup to give the same taste, with fewer calories. Make sure to get good quality Gruyere and use a cheese planer for a super-thin slice.

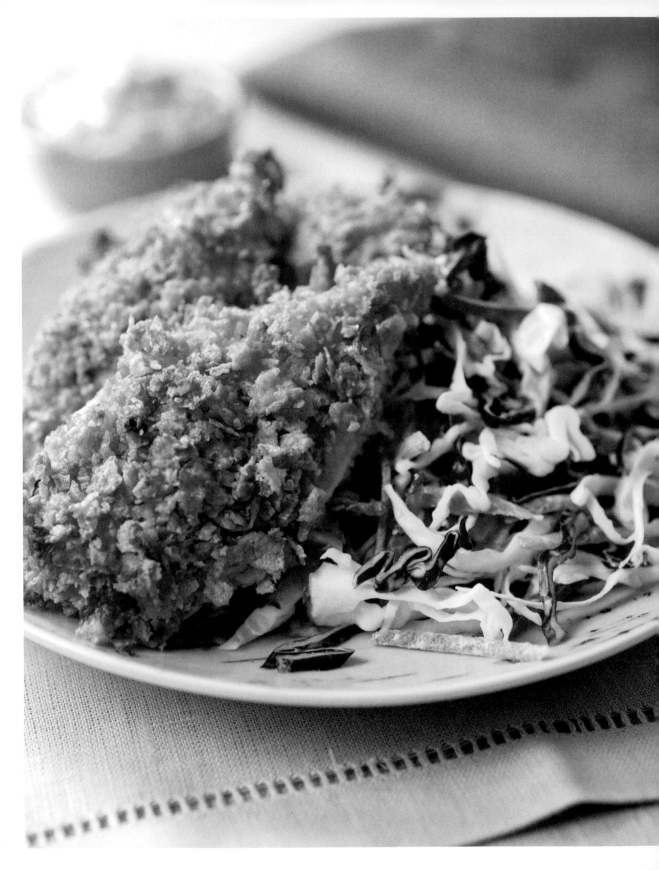

Oven-Baked Crispy Chicken Tenders with Coleslaw

Cornflakes give oven-"fried" chicken the crunchy crust we like, without the fat of frying, or sautéing. Marinating the chicken for an hour in a buttermilk marinade, with garlic and herbs, really boosts the flavor. The half-buttermilk / half low-fat sour cream "mayonnaise" is a slimmer innovation you can bring to lots of other dishes.

SERVES 4
Calories per serving, chicken with coleslaw: 519
Calories per serving, tartar sauce: 27

For the chicken:
2 cloves garlic, smashed
1/4 teaspoon dried thyme
1 bay leaf
2 teaspoons salt
1/4 teaspoon red pepper flakes
1/2 cup nonfat buttermilk
1 pound chicken tenders (about 12)
1 1/2 cups cornflakes, crushed to medium crumbs
    Nonstick cooking spray

For the tartar sauce:
1 1/2 tablespoons low-fat sour cream
1 tablespoon nonfat buttermilk
    Juice of 1/2 lemon
1/4 cup fresh parsley leaves, chopped
1 tablespoon drained nonpareil capers
1 tablespoon chopped sweet gherkin
1 tablespoon water

For the coleslaw:
1 1/2 (10 ounce bags) cabbage slaw mix
1 red bell pepper, sliced thin
2 tablespoons thin-sliced red onion
2 tablespoons shredded fresh basil leaves, plus whole leaves, for garnish
2 tablespoons shredded fresh mint, plus whole leaves, for garnish
1 tablespoon low-fat sour cream
1 tablespoon nonfat buttermilk
1 tablespoon seasoned rice wine vinegar
2–3 dashes hot pepper sauce
1/8 teaspoon salt
1/8 teaspoon pepper
8 cherry tomatoes, quartered, for garnish

1. PREHEAT the oven to 400 degrees. Line a baking sheet with aluminum foil and spray lightly with cooking spray. Set aside.

2. FOR THE CHICKEN: In a medium bowl, combine the garlic, spices, and buttermilk. Add the chicken and turn in the marinade. Cover and refrigerate 1 hour.

3. FOR THE COLESLAW: In a large bowl, combine the cabbage slaw mix, bell pepper, onion, and shredded herbs. In a separate smaller bowl, whisk together the sour cream, buttermilk, vinegar, hot pepper sauce, salt, and pepper. Pour the dressing over the vegetables and toss to coat.

4. FOR THE TARTAR SAUCE: Whisk together all of the ingredients in a separate small bowl.

5. PLACE the cornflake crumbs on a plate. Drain the chicken tenders. Pick up a chicken tender with one hand, and turn it in the cornflake coating, using the other hand to gently press additional coating onto the sides. Place on the prepared baking sheet. Continue on in this way to coat all of the chicken pieces, arranging them on the baking sheet in a single layer. Bake at 400 degrees until firm, about 15 minutes.

6. TO SERVE, divide the coleslaw between 4 bowls. Arrange 3 chicken tenders, standing up with wide ends at the bottom and overlapping slightly, at one side of each mound. Drizzle the sauce over the chicken. Garnish bowls with chopped cherry tomatoes, and fresh herbs.

Chicken Caesar Salad

We've always loved this classic salad, and we love it even more now that it's been spruced-up so well. Arugula, seared chicken breast, and nutty sunflower seeds, plus the nearly fat-free yogurt and mustard dressing really gives this dinner salad bite. A soft boiled egg is an indulgent touch!

SERVES 2
Calories per serving: 445

For the salad:

   8-ounce chicken breast, skinless
   A little olive oil to brush onto the chicken
4 thin (melba thin) slices baguette on the diagonal
   A little olive oil to brush onto the toast before crisping in hot oven
$\frac{1}{2}$ medium garlic clove
2 heads baby romaine lettuce
1 soft-boiled, large, free-range egg, at room temperature
   One handful of arugula and mustard cress
2 tablespoons finely grated Parmesan
1 tablespoon sunflower seeds

For the dressing:

2 tablespoons fat-free Greek yogurt
   The other $\frac{1}{2}$ garlic clove
1 teaspoon Dijon mustard
1 teaspoon malt vinegar
1 tablespoon olive oil
   salt and black pepper

1. PREHEAT oven to 350 degrees.

2. BRUSH the chicken with a little olive oil.

3. ON A HOT GRILL PAN, sear the chicken breast for 4 to 5 minutes before flipping over and doing the same on the other side.

4. WHILE THE CHICKEN IS SEARING, prepare the baguette toasts. Slice the baguette on the diagonal and place on a baking sheet. Brush on a little olive oil. Toast the bread for about 10 minutes, until crisp. Rub with the garlic clove.

5. ONCE YOU HAVE STRONG GRILL MARKS over the chicken breast on both sides, cover your pan with foil and place into the hot oven on the higher shelf for 15 minutes.

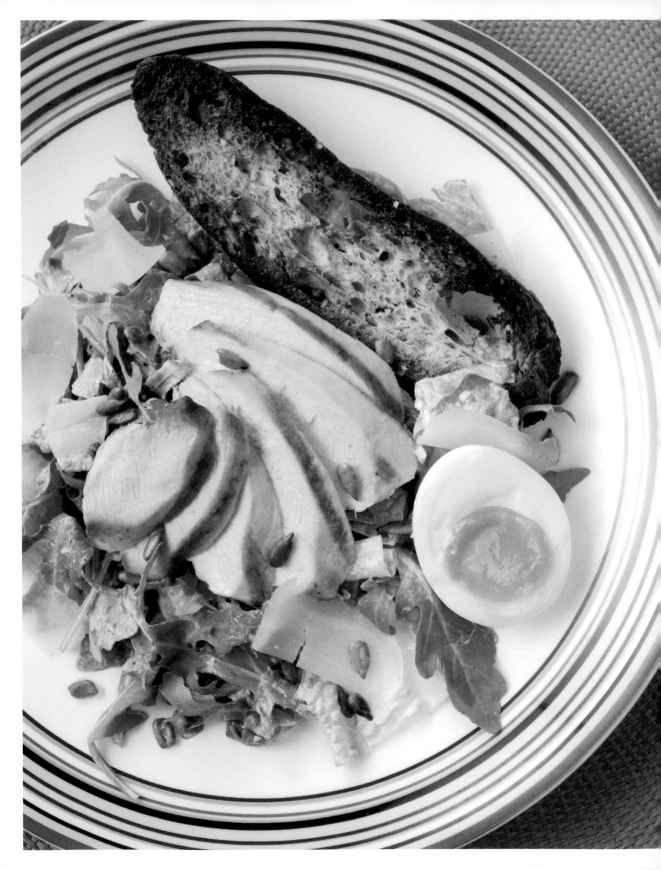

6. MEANWHILE, wash the lettuce and spin dry.

7. CAREFULLY DROP the egg in boiling water for 5 minutes exactly. Empty the boiling water out of the pan and replace it with cold water. Let the egg stand in the cold water while you finish the recipe.

8. TO MAKE THE DRESSING, combine all the ingredients into a small mixing bowl and stir together with a whisk. Taste and season before setting aside.

9. PUT the washed and dried salad leaves into a big bowl with the dressing. Toss for a couple of minutes to make sure that all the leaves are coated. Add the shaved/grated Parmesan and arugula. Toss once again.

10. REMOVE the chicken from the oven and let it cool down enough to handle before slicing on the diagonal.

11. PLATE UP THE SALAD, making sure that the chicken is evenly distributed.

12. TUCK the crispy baguette toasts on the side of the salad and add half a soft-boiled egg. Finally grind over some black pepper, scatter the sunflower seeds, and serve.

Spinach and Mushroom Veggie Lasagna

This indulgent three-layer vegetable lasagna redefines delicious. We added sautéed mushrooms in place of the ground beef, and cut calories by removing half the mozzarella cheese, but keeping it where you'll taste it most—as a gooey top layer. Plus, we've added plenty of fresh basil, oregano, and thyme, adding vivid flavor without the fat.

MAKES 12 SERVINGS
Calories per serving: 337

2   tablespoons olive oil
1½   pounds cremini and/or shiitake mushrooms, sliced
1   teaspoon dried thyme
     Kosher salt
1   15-ounce container part-skim ricotta
¾   cup skim milk
2   eggs, lightly beaten
3   cups shredded, part-skim mozzarella cheese, divided evenly
¾   cup grated Parmesan cheese
1   10-ounce box frozen chopped spinach, defrosted and drained
⅓   cup chopped fresh basil, plus more to garnish
1   teaspoon dried oregano
     Freshly ground black pepper
5   cups tomato sauce
12   sheets no-cook lasagna noodles
     Nonstick cooking spray

1. PREHEAT the oven to 375 degrees.

2. HEAT the olive oil in a large skillet over medium-high heat. Add the mushrooms and thyme and season with salt. Cook until softened, about 10 to 12 minutes.

3. IN A MEDIUM BOWL, combine the ricotta, milk, and eggs and stir. Add 1 cup of mozzarella, Parmesan, spinach, basil and oregano; season with salt and pepper and stir to incorporate.

4. SPREAD 1 cup of tomato sauce in the bottom of a 9-by-13-by-2-inch pan. Layer 4 sheets of lasagna on top, slightly overlapping. Spread half the ricotta mixture on the noodles, and cover with half the mushroom

mixture. Top with 1½ cups tomato sauce. Repeat with 4 sheets of lasagna pasta, remaining ricotta mixture, remaining mushrooms, and 1½ cups tomato sauce. Cover with the remaining 4 sheets of lasagna, the remaining cup of tomato sauce, and the remaining mozzarella cheese.

5. LIGHTLY COAT a sheet of aluminum foil with nonstick spray and cover the uncooked lasagna, spray-side down. Bake at 375 degrees, covered, until bubbly, about 45 minutes. Remove foil from lasagna and increase the oven temperature to 450 degrees. Cook until cheese browns, about 12 minutes. Remove from the oven and let stand for 15 minutes before cutting. Serve warm and garnish with basil.

Tip

To lower the calories, reduce the mozzarella to 2 cups and the grated Parmesan to ¾ cup.

Pasta Bake with Sausage, Broccoli, and Beans

Turkey sausage trims down this classic Italian combination, while beans deliver protein and fiber. Make it deliciously creamy and tangy with skim milk ricotta and tangy Pecorino.

SERVES 8
Calories per serving: 529

½   teaspoon salt
1   large head of broccoli, about 1½ pounds, cut into small florets
3   cloves garlic, peeled
¾   pound rigatoni
1   tablespoon olive oil, plus more for pan
1   pound Italian-style turkey sausage with fennel
    (removed from casing if uncooked, or sliced thinly if precooked)
1   can cannellini or great northern beans, rinsed and drained
⅔   pound of skim mozzarella, grated, ¼ cup reserved
¾   cup skim ricotta cheese
½   cup chicken stock
½   cup Pecorino Romano cheese, finely grated, ¼ cup reserved
1   teaspoon salt
½   teaspoon ground pepper
3   tablespoons breadcrumbs
1   tablespoon olive oil

1. PREHEAT oven to 375 degrees. Lightly oil a 9-by-13-inch gratin or baking dish.

2. IN A SEPARATE POT, bring water to a boil and add ½ teaspoon of salt, broccoli, and garlic. Simmer the broccoli and garlic for 5 minutes, until softened. With a slotted spoon remove the broccoli and garlic to a large bowl. Bring the water back to the boil, add the pasta, and cook the pasta for about 2 minutes less than the package directions suggest, about 11 minutes. The pasta should be al dente, a little firm.

3. MEANWHILE, in a large dutch oven set over medium high heat, heat the oil. Add sausage and the garlic cloves from the broccoli bowl, and cook, stirring frequently until meat is fully cooked and no longer pink, about 4 to 5 minutes, if using fresh sausage. (If using fully cooked sausage

cook until surface is golden, about 2 to 3 minutes.) With a slotted spoon, transfer sausage to the broccoli, and drain most of oil from the pan, leaving about 2 tablespoons. Discard the garlic.

4. TOSS drained pasta with sausage mixture. Add beans, stock, ¾ cup of grated mozzarella cheese, and all of the ricotta. Add remaining salt and pepper. Gently toss. Transfer to prepared gratin or baking dish, top with breadcrumbs, remaining ¼ cup of grated cheese and ¼ cup mozzarella cheese and drizzle with olive oil.

5. IF MAKING THIS IN ADVANCE, allow the mixture to come to room temperature, cover with plastic wrap and place in the refrigerator.

6. BAKE for 25 minutes, until heated through and crusty on top.

Tips

1. Be careful not to use breakfast sausage. If you can't find Italian style sausage, you can add 1/4 teaspoon of fennel seeds to the pan while you cook the sausage.

2. If you want to reduce the calories, you can remove the beans.

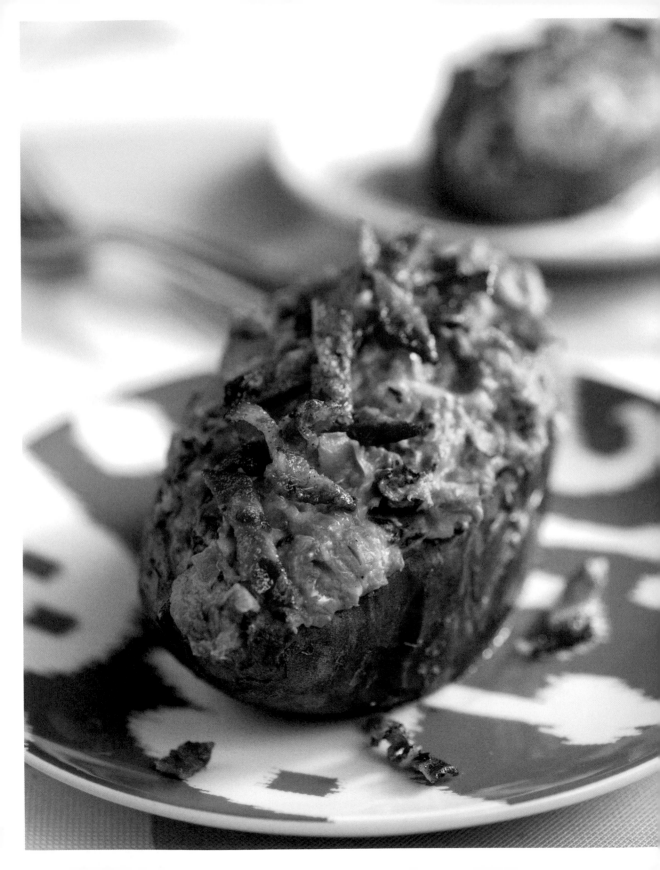

Healthy Potato Skins

No one's ever accused potato skins of being healthy—until now! Turkey bacon, spinach, and nutty, nutritious sweet potatoes are the stars in this low-fat version of the greatest snack food ever.

SERVES 2
Calories per serving: 420

2	medium sweet potatoes
1	teaspoon olive oil
1	small onion, diced
1	clove garlic, minced
1	bag baby spinach (about 9 ounces)
2	scallions, thinly sliced
2	slices turkey bacon
4	ounces low-fat cream cheese
¼	cup low-fat buttermilk
1	teaspoon salt
¼	teaspoon freshly ground black pepper
1	teaspoon vegetable oil
2	tablespoons grated Parmesan cheese

1. PREHEAT the oven to 350 degrees.

2. PLACE sweet potatoes on a baking sheet and onto an oven rack. Bake at 350 degrees for 45 minutes or until fork tender.

3. MEANWHILE, in a deep sauté pan heat the olive oil and cook the onion for 2 to 3 minutes until soft. Add the garlic and cook for one more minute. Add the entire bag of spinach and scallions, cover, and cook 3 to 4 minutes until the spinach has wilted.

4. IN ANOTHER SAUTÉ PAN cook the turkey bacon until crisp and transfer to a plate lined with paper towels to drain. When cooled, chop the bacon into small pieces and reserve.

5. WHEN THE SWEET POTATOES ARE COOKED, let them cool for 5 minutes. Carefully slice each one in half and scoop out inside of potato into a bowl. Add cream cheese, buttermilk, salt, and pepper and mash together until smooth.

6. USING A PASTRY BRUSH, coat the outside of each potato skin with the vegetable oil. Fill each of the shells with the filling and top with a sprinkle of Parmesan cheese. Transfer each skin back to the baking sheet and cook for 15 to 20 minutes or until the top is golden brown and the skins are crispy. Top with bits of turkey bacon and serve.

Tip

Quarter the potatoes to serve as a starter or light snack.

Easy Herb-Roasted Chicken with Roasted Veggies

It's hard to imagine a more satisfying meal than roasted chicken and vegetables, and this version—with its fragrant chicken, red and golden beets, and an optional tantalizing drizzle of heady white truffle oil—just might be the best version of all.

SERVES 4
Calories per serving: 403

For the roasted chicken:
1   3.5- to 4-pound whole chicken
1   clove garlic, minced
1   tablespoon fresh thyme leaves, chopped
1   tablespoon fresh sage, chopped
2   tablespoons fresh rosemary, chopped
    Rosemary stems
    Salt, to taste
    Pepper, to taste
2   tablespoons olive oil
1   lemon, sliced

For the roasted root vegetables:
¼   pound golden beets, peeled and stems trimmed
¼   pound red beets, peeled and stems trimmed
¼   pound whole baby carrots, peeled and stems trimmed
2   tablespoons olive oil
1   tablespoon white truffle oil
    Salt, to taste
    Pepper, to taste
1   teaspoon fresh rosemary
1   teaspoon fresh thyme

1. PREHEAT the oven to 475 degrees.

2. WASH the chicken and pat dry with paper towels. Season the cavity with salt and season the outside of the chicken with salt and pepper.

3. IN A BOWL, mix together the garlic, thyme, sage, rosemary, and olive oil. Rub into the cavity of the chicken as well as the outside.

4. PLACE the rosemary stems inside the cavity and squeeze the lemon juice inside as well. Leave the slices inside and place the chicken in a roasting pan. Cook in the oven at 475 degrees for 1 to 1½ hours or until the chicken is golden brown and the juices run clear. Remove from the oven and let sit for 10 minutes before carving.

5. TO MAKE THE ROASTED ROOT VEGETABLES: Place the vegetables in a large mixing bowl and season with salt and pepper. Drizzle with the olive

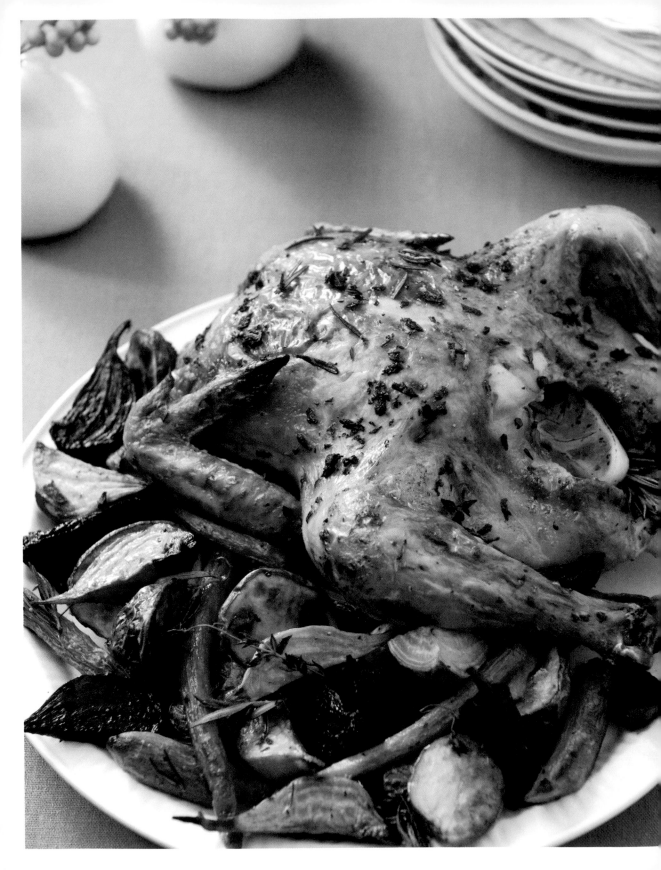

oil and an optional drizzle of white truffle oil and place in a roasting pan or on a baking sheet. Sprinkle the fresh herbs over the vegetables and roast in the oven for 45 minutes, turning once halfway through the cooking time. Serve with the roast chicken.

Tip

Truffle oil is costly, but a little goes a long way to add a deep heady fragrance to potatoes or pasta.

Pasta Primavera

We say bring on the veggies in this gorgeous pasta dish. Asparagus and scallions bring a hint of spring to balance out a medley of earthy mushrooms.

SERVES 4
Calories per serving: 445

3/4 pound standard, whole wheat, or whole grain penne
1 pound (1 bunch) medium asparagus, tough bottom stems broken off and discarded, remainder cut into 1 1/2-inch sections
1 (15-ounce) can chicken stock
1/4 teaspoon salt
Pepper, to taste
1 1/2 tablespoons, plus 2 teaspoons olive oil
4 cloves garlic, sliced
1/4 red onion, chopped small
1/8 teaspoon red pepper flakes
4 ounces shiitake mushrooms, stemmed and sliced
4 ounces cremini mushrooms, trimmed and cut into quarters or sixths, depending on size
1 cup frozen peas
2 pieces sun-dried tomatoes
2 tablespoons chopped fresh parsley
1/2 cup grated Parmesan cheese
6-ounce bag baby spinach
2 scallions, chopped

1. BRING a large pot of salted water to a boil for the pasta.

2. COMBINE the asparagus, 1/4 cup of stock, and 1/4 teaspoon salt in a large skillet. Cover, and cook over medium heat, until al dente, 3 to 5 minutes. Transfer to a bowl with any remaining stock. Set aside.

3. IN THE SAME SKILLET, heat the oil with the garlic and onion over low heat. Cover and cook until the vegetables soften but do not brown, 3 to 4 minutes. Stir in the red pepper flakes. Add the mushrooms, and raise the heat to medium-high. Cook until the mushrooms are lightly browned and softened, about 5 minutes. If mushrooms begin to stick to the bottom of the pan, add 2 tablespoons stock and stir to release. Add the peas, the rest of the stock, and 1 tablespoon of the parsley. Remove from the heat and set aside.

4. ADD the pasta to the boiling water and cook about two-thirds of the way, about 6 minutes.

5. REMOVE 1 cup of pasta water and add it to the skillet with the vegetables. Drain the pasta in a colander, and add it to the skillet. Bring liquid to a boil; cook until reduced by about one-half. Add all but about 2 tablespoons of the Parmesan cheese, the asparagus, $\frac{1}{2}$ teaspoon salt, $\frac{1}{4}$ teaspoon pepper, and the spinach. Cook, tossing with tongs, until the liquid is reduced and thickened and the spinach is wilted, 1 to 2 minutes.

6. DIVIDE the pasta between 4 bowls, and sprinkle with scallions and sun-dried tomatoes. Drizzle each with $\frac{1}{2}$ teaspoon oil, and sprinkle with the remaining cheese.

Tips

1. You can make a pasta sauce with very little fat by boiling canned chicken stock with a little olive oil, grated cheese, and some of the pasta cooking water. The starch from the pasta water thickens the sauce as it reduces.

2. The pasta cooks partway on its own, then finishes cooking in the skillet with the vegetables and sauce. The pasta will pick up the flavors of the veggies and sauce as it finishes in the skillet.

Turkey Chili Crunch

Southwestern flavors and a hint of cocoa blend with dynamic results in this chili we whip up for all our casual get-togethers. Ground turkey masquerades as beef with a fraction of the fat and the illusion continues with fat-free yogurt cooling the chipotle instead of sour cream.

SERVES 6
Calories per serving: 355

1	tablespoon olive oil
1	pound ground turkey
	Salt
	Pepper
2	teaspoons chili powder
1	teaspoon ground cumin
1	teaspoon dried oregano
	Pinch ground cinnamon
1/2	red onion, chopped (about 1 cup)
3	cloves garlic, chopped
2	carrots, diced (1/2 inch), about 1 cup
1	can (14-ounce) chopped whole tomatoes, with juice
1/2	chipotle pepper in adobo, seeded and chopped, with about 1/2 teaspoon adobo sauce
3	cups water
1	tablespoon cocoa powder
2	(14- to 15-ounce) cans pinto beans, drained and rinsed
1/2	cup chopped cilantro (leaves and slender stems), plus 1/4 cup for serving
	Bittersweet chocolate, grated, for serving
3	scallions, chopped, for serving
1/2	cup nonfat yogurt, for serving
	Tortilla chips, for garnish

1. IN A LARGE, heavy-bottomed saucepan, heat the oil over medium heat. Add the turkey, 1/2 teaspoon salt, and 1/4 teaspoon pepper and cook, stirring, 3 minutes. Add the chili powder, cumin, oregano, and cinnamon, and cook, stirring, 3 minutes, or until the water evaporates and the turkey sizzles.

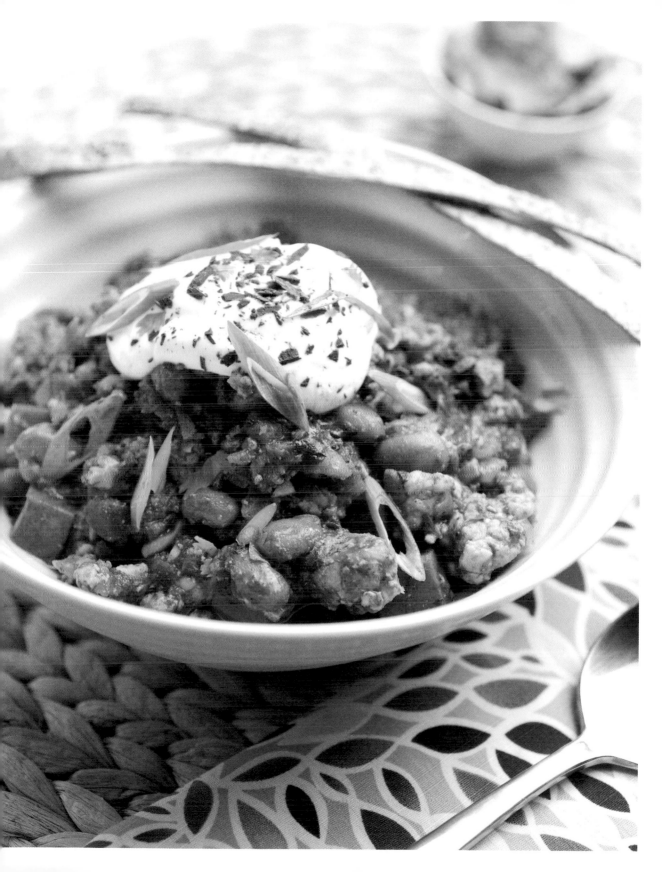

2. ADD the onion, garlic, and ½ teaspoon salt. Cover and cook until the onion is wilted, 5 to 7 minutes. If the onion or the spices begin to stick to the pan, add 2 tablespoons water and scrape with a wooden spoon to release.

3. ADD the carrots, tomatoes, chipotle pepper, water, and cocoa powder. Bring to a simmer, reduce the heat to low, and cook, partially covered, 25 minutes. Stir in the beans and ½ cup cilantro and cook 15 more minutes.

4. SPRAY a whole wheat tortilla with cooking spray and season with salt and pepper (or cayenne and ground cumin). Slice thinly and bake in a preheated 400 degree oven for 5–10 minutes until crispy.

5. TO SERVE, ladle into soup bowls and grate a tiny amount of chocolate over each. Top with scallions, the remaining cilantro, a spoonful of yogurt, and some grated chocolate! Garnish with tortilla chips.

Scrumptious Skinny Spaghetti and Meatballs

Meatballs are as versatile as they are classic, either with pasta and sauce, on toasted whole grain bread for a sandwich or even on their own served with a dash of chutney. You limit the fat by choosing lean meats. You're in control.

SERVES 4
Calories per serving: 560

2	12-ounce to 14-ounce jars of your favorite marinara sauce
2	slices of your favorite sandwich bread
$3/4$	cup water
$1/3$	pound ground veal
$1/3$	pound ground pork
$1/3$	pound ground turkey
$1/2$	cup grated Parmesan cheese, plus more for serving
1	large egg
$1/2$	small onion, finely minced
$1/3$	cup chopped parsley
2	tablespoons chopped basil
1	teaspoon oregano
1	teaspoon salt
$1/4$	teaspoon red pepper flakes
8	ounces whole wheat spaghetti

1. HEAT marinara sauce in a large, wide pot over medium heat. Cover to prevent splattering.

2. REMOVE crusts from bread, place bread in a medium bowl and pour water over. Let sit 10 minutes, and gently squeeze out excess liquid. Put bread in a large bowl, discard water.

3. ADD all the ground meats, cheese, egg, onion, parsley, basil, oregano, salt, and red pepper flakes to bowl with bread. Gently toss to combine, maintaining a light touch to keep air in the meatballs (don't squish the meat too much, or you'll end up with tough meatballs). Roll the meat mixture in your hands to create meatballs slightly larger than a golf ball.

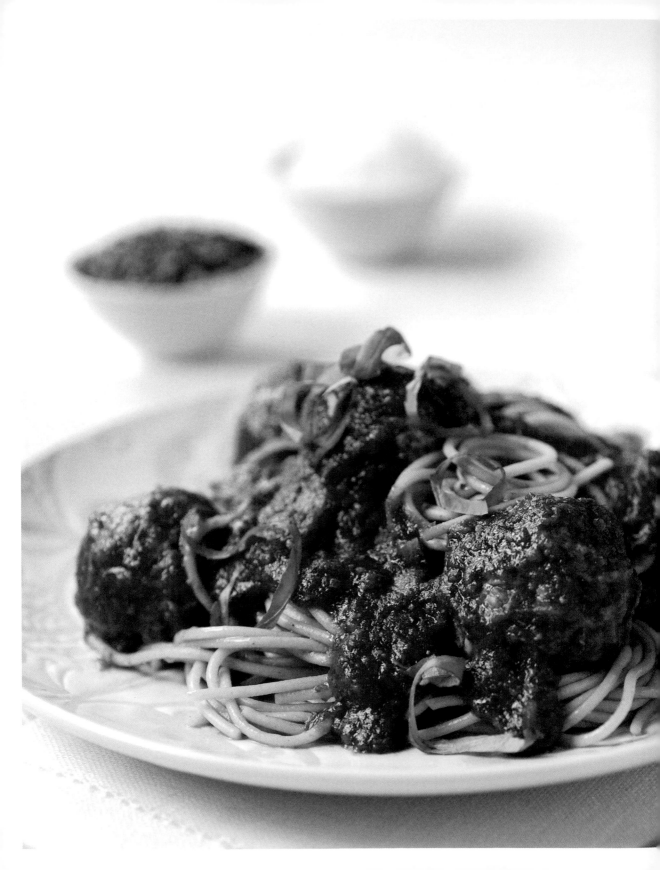

4. REMOVE marinara sauce from heat to prevent splattering, gently drop the meatballs in the warm sauce. Return tomato sauce to medium-low heat, bring to a simmer and cook, covered, until meatballs have cooked through, about 30 minutes.

5. COOK pasta according to package, toss with marinara sauce, and top with meatballs.

Tip

Make your own marinara. Heat 1 tablespoon olive oil and sauté 2 cloves minced garlic until lightly golden. Add 32 ounces of canned, peeled, crushed plum tomatoes and simmer for 10 minutes. Add meatballs, 2 tablespoons of torn fresh basil leaves, and season with $1\frac{1}{2}$ teaspoons salt and $\frac{1}{2}$ teaspoon pepper. Cook for 30 minutes.

Mushroom and Spinach Quiche with Potato Crust

Elevate your lunch to a whole new level with our creative spin on quiche. A crunchy potato crust replaces the traditional butter laden pastry shell, leaving you with just as much flavor, but far fewer calories! We like to fill ours with a healthy dose of veggies and sprinkle of cheese, but you can adapt this recipe to suit just about any palate. Serve with a side salad and enjoy!

SERVES 8
Calories per serving: 210

$\frac{1}{2}$	pound Yukon Gold potatoes, peeled and shredded
$3\frac{1}{4}$	teaspoons olive oil
$\frac{1}{2}$	teaspoon salt
$\frac{1}{2}$	teaspoon pepper
1	onion, diced
8	ounces white mushrooms, sliced
	5-ounce bag baby spinach
3	large eggs
1	cup skim milk
1	ounce Gruyere or cheddar cheese, shredded in a food processor, or on the large holes of a grater

1. PREHEAT oven to 400 degrees.

2. LIGHTLY GREASE a 9-inch glass or ceramic pie dish with $\frac{1}{4}$ teaspoon oil. Toss potatoes with 1 teaspoon oil and $\frac{1}{8}$ teaspoon each salt and pepper. Press into an even layer in a pie dish, up the sides like a crust. Bake until golden brown at the edges and dry, about 20 minutes. Let cool.

3. LOWER THE OVEN to 325 degrees. Heat 1 teaspoon oil in a large skillet, preferably nonstick, over medium heat. Add onion and cook until softened and golden, about 5 minutes. Add remaining teaspoon oil and mushrooms and cook, stirring, until mushrooms release their liquid and most of the liquid evaporates, about 8 minutes. Add spinach and $\frac{1}{4}$ teaspoon each salt and pepper, and cook, stirring, just until spinach wilts, about 30 seconds. Let cool slightly.

4. WHISK together eggs, milk, and remaining $\frac{1}{8}$ teaspoon salt and pepper. Spread the mushroom mixture in an even layer in the pie dish, and top with an even layer of the cheese. Carefully pour in egg mixture. Bake until firm around the edges, but still wobbly in the center, about 20 minutes. Let cool, and serve warm or at room temperature.

Tips

1. Make individual quiches by using muffin tins.

2. Feel free to experiment with your favorite vegetables like broccoli, asparagus, or red peppers.

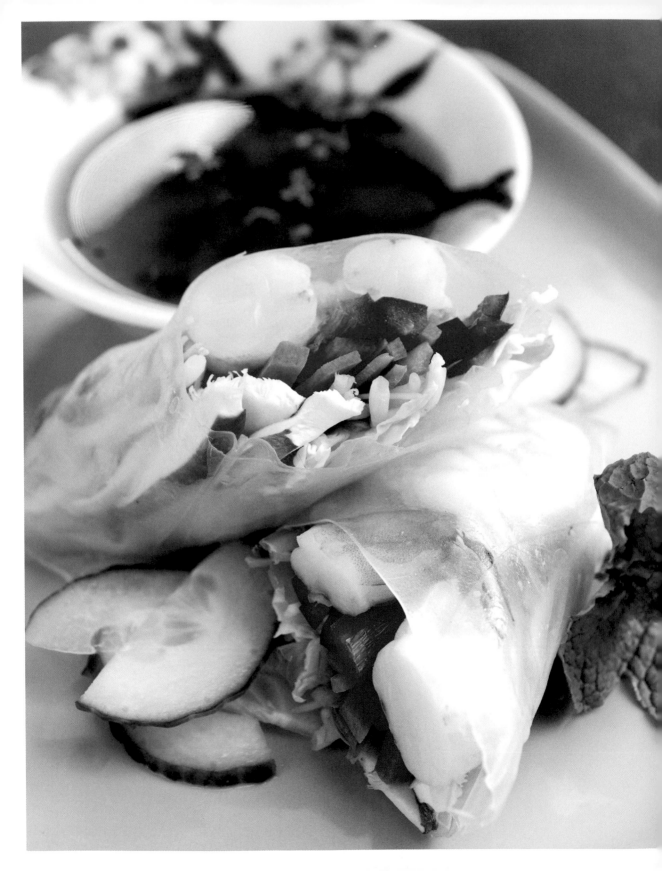

Spring Rolls with Lemongrass Dipping Sauce and Cucumber Salad

Low-fat and delicious come naturally to the dynamic flavors of Southeast Asia, and these spring rolls with lemongrass dipping sauce make that abundantly clear. It's a festival of fresh as shrimp and veggies get to show off amid garlic, ginger, mint, and bright rice vinegar.

MAKES 6 ROLLS
Calories per serving, 2 spring rolls: 104
Calories per serving, lemongrass dipping sauce: 63
Calories per serving, cucumber salad: 39

For the lemongrass dipping sauce:

½ cup rice vinegar
½ cup honey
1 stalk lemongrass, minced
2 garlic cloves, minced
1 tablespoon ginger, minced
1 teaspoon red chili flakes

For the cucumber salad:

1 English (hothouse) cucumber
1 tablespoon mirin
1 tablespoon sesame oil
1 tablespoon rice vinegar
Salt, to taste

For the spring rolls:

1 tablespoon sesame oil
1 tablespoon ginger, minced
1 tablespoon garlic, minced
½ pound medium shrimp
(about 12 to 13)
1 tablespoon mirin
1 tablespoon soy sauce

For the assembly:

6 Vietnamese rice paper wraps, soaked in cold water for 50 seconds
2 ounces red bell pepper, julienne
½ large carrot, shredded (about 2 ounces)
2 cups bean sprouts
2 ounces sugar snap peas, julienne
Reserved shrimp, from above
2 ounces shiitake mushrooms, thinly sliced
6 teaspoons mint, chiffonade (shredded), for garnish
2 tablespoons scallions, green parts only, sliced on the bias, for garnish

1. FOR THE LEMONGRASS DIPPING SAUCE: In a small stainless steel saucepan over medium heat, combine the rice vinegar and honey. Bring to a boil and reduce to a simmer. Cook for about 10 to 15 minutes or until it reaches a syrupy consistency. Remove from the heat and add the minced garlic, ginger, and chili flakes and let steep until cooled, about another 30 minutes. Set aside and reserve.

2. FOR THE CUCUMBER SALAD: Wash and cut the English (hothouse) cucumber in half, lengthwise. Slice into thin half-moons and transfer to a bowl.

3. IN A SEPARATE SMALLER BOWL, whisk together the mirin, sesame oil, and rice vinegar. Season to taste with salt. Drizzle the dressing over the sliced cucumber and toss. Refrigerate until ready to serve.

4. FOR THE SHRIMP: Over medium to high heat, place the sesame oil, minced ginger, garlic, and the shrimp. Cook until the shrimp are pink and not too firm. Add the mirin and let it reduce. Add the soy sauce and cook another minute. Let cool and set aside.

5. FOR THE ASSEMBLY: Soak the rice wrappers in cold water for 45 seconds or until pliable. Be careful not to rip the wrappers when removing from the water. Place on cutting board lined with a clean dish towel and spread evenly.

6. PLACE some red bell pepper strips, shredded carrots, bean sprouts, shiitake mushrooms, sugar snap peas, two reserved shrimp, and 1 teaspoon of shredded mint on each wrapper. Start wrapping at one end and roll over once, then bring in both ends and continue to roll making sure the filling remains inside and fits snugly. Continue with remaining wrappers and filling.

7. CUT each spring roll on the bias and serve with the cucumber salad and the lemongrass dipping sauce. Garnish with sliced scallions.

Sesame Peanut Noodles

Sesame noodles are always on our minds when we order in Chinese food, so we gave this Asian mainstay a makeover by adding slaw and jicama to bring in the crunch.

SERVES 6
Calories per serving: 308

For the noodles:
8   ounces whole wheat spaghetti

For the dressing:
2   tablespoons rice vinegar
1/4 cup low-sodium soy sauce
1/4 cup peanut butter
2   tablespoons grated ginger
1   tablespoon dark sesame oil
1   teaspoon brown sugar
   Juice of one lime
1/2 cup water, hot

For the assembly:
1/2 bag store-bought coleslaw mix
1/2 cup red pepper
1/2 cup cilantro, chopped
1/2 a lime, squeezed
1/2 cup apple
1/2 cup jicama
1   teaspoon toasted sesame seeds
2   scallions, julienne

For the garnish:
1/2 cup dry-roasted peanuts,
   for garnish
   Cilantro, chopped
   Lime wedges

1. BRING a pot of water to a boil for the pasta and cook the pasta according to package instructions. Drain and run under cold water.

2. TO MAKE THE DRESSING, combine all the ingredients into a small mixing bowl and stir together with a whisk. Add the dressing to the pasta and toss. Stir in the coleslaw mix, red pepper, and cilantro. Squeeze a half of a lime over and toss.

3. ADD the remaining ingredients, toss and refrigerate for one hour. Garnish with dry-roasted peanuts, chopped cilantro, and lime wedges. Serve.

Chicken and Bean Burritos with Pineapple Salsa

Juicy poached chicken and lots of veggies stuff this smart burrito full of flavor without maxing out your calories. Top it off with a squirt of lime and some low-fat cheese, and dig in.

SERVES 4

Calories per serving, chicken and bean burritos: 436
Calories per serving, pineapple salsa: 28

For the chicken and bean burritos:

1   cup fresh or frozen corn kernels, thawed and drained, if frozen
1   (15 1/2-ounce) can black beans, drained and rinsed
1/2   cup fresh cilantro leaves, chopped
1 1/2   tablespoons fresh lime juice
1   teaspoon minced fresh jalapeño (optional)
1/4   teaspoon salt
1/8   teaspoon cayenne pepper
3/4   pound bone-in, skin-on split chicken breasts
3   peppercorns
1   carrot, sliced
1   bay leaf
3   medium tomatoes, 2 quartered, 1 diced
1   white onion, quartered
6   garlic cloves
1 1/2   teaspoons vegetable oil
4   medium flour tortillas
1/4   cup shredded low-fat cheddar
1/4   cup shredded iceberg lettuce

For the pineapple salsa:

1   cup ripe pineapple, chopped
1/4   cup red onions, chopped
1/4   cup roasted red bell pepper, chopped
1   tablespoon fresh cilantro, chopped
1   tablespoon fresh lime juice

1. HEAT a medium skillet over medium heat. Add the corn and cook, shaking the pan occasionally, until browned, about 5 minutes. Transfer to a medium bowl. Add beans, cilantro, lime, jalapeño, salt, and cayenne, and stir until well mixed; set aside.

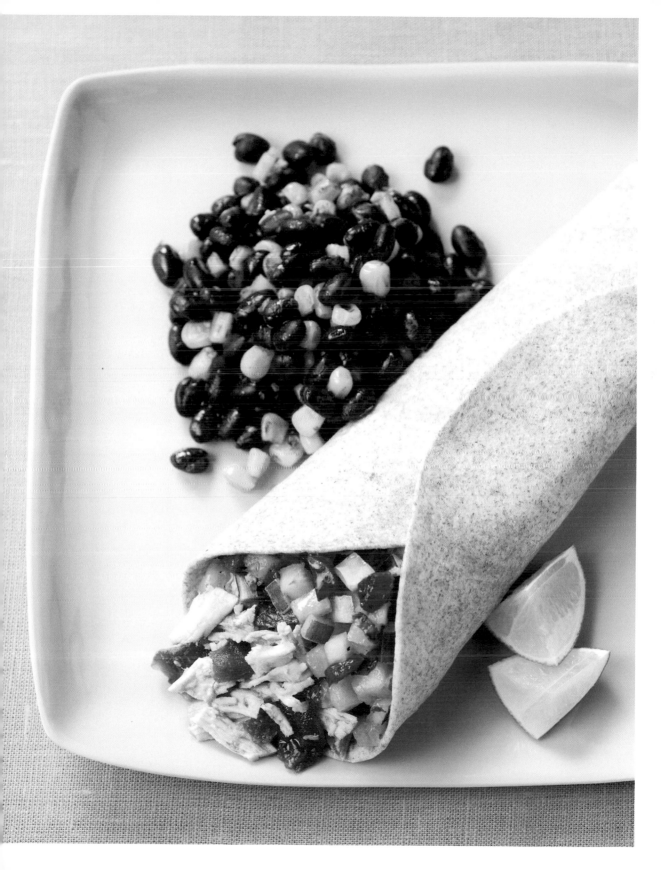

2. PUT the chicken, peppercorns, carrot, bay leaf, and 3 of the garlic cloves in a large saucepan and add enough water to cover by 2 inches. Bring to a boil, then simmer over medium heat until cooked through, about 25 minutes. Let cool slightly in the broth. Remove the chicken from the broth, and remove the skin and bones. Shred the chicken into small pieces, and return the meat to the broth.

3. PUT the quartered tomatoes, onion, and garlic in a blender and blend until smooth. Heat the oil in a large, deep skillet over medium-high heat. Add the tomato mixture and cook, stirring until thickened and fragrant, about 5 minutes. Using a slotted spoon, transfer the shredded chicken to the tomato mixture. Stir until well mixed.

4. HEAT a large skillet over medium heat. Warm the tortillas, one at a time, until pliable, about 1 minute. Divide the cheese, lettuce, diced tomato, bean mixture, and chicken with its sauce among the tortillas, spreading the ingredients in a line down the center. Fold in the top and bottom, then roll in the sides. Serve immediately.

5. TO MAKE THE PINEAPPLE SALSA: Place all the ingredients in a bowl and mix together. Set aside.

Tips

1. Poaching is a traditional low-fat method for cooking lean chicken breasts; once poached, the meat is shredded and returned to the poaching broth to keep chicken moist.

2. Swap the high-calorie chips and salsa for this tangy, pineapple salsa. Making it in advance will allow the fruit to macerate with the juice.

3. Instead of salty, fatty chips, reach for baked chips, jicama, or radish slices. Also try with roast chicken, grilled pork tenderloin, or fish.

Ultimate Sausage Cheese Pizza

This personal pie gets its pizzeria credentials from roasted red peppers, basil-flecked chicken sausage, and a sprinkle of Parmesan cheese.

SERVES 1
Calories per serving: 475

1	teaspoon olive oil
¼	tablespoon minced garlic
¼	cup organic tomato sauce
⅛	teaspoon salt
	Pinch pepper
1	chicken basil sausage link precooked
	Salt, to taste
	Pepper, to taste
½	red bell pepper—jarred roasted red peppers work and are a great time-saver
4	ounces prepared pizza dough
2	tablespoons shredded Parmesan cheese
1	tablespoon chopped scallion, white and green parts
1	teaspoon coarsely chopped fresh basil (optional)

1. PREHEAT the oven to 450 degrees.

2. FOR THE TOMATO SAUCE, heat oil in a small saucepan over medium heat, add garlic and cook for 1 minute. Add tomato sauce, salt, and pepper and simmer for 4 to 5 minutes.

3. PREHEAT a gas grill or stovetop grill pan over medium high heat. Place chicken basil sausage and bell pepper on the grill. Grill the sausage until cooked through, about 2 minutes each side; set aside. Continue grilling the pepper, turning, until the skin is blackened, 10 to 15 minutes.

4. PLACE pepper in a bowl, cover with plastic wrap, and let stand until cool enough to handle. Peel, stem, and seed the pepper; cut or tear half the pepper into large dice, reserve the other half roasted pepper for another dish. When chicken sausage is done slice thinly and set aside.

5. SPRAY an aluminum pizza pan with nonfat cooking spray. On a lightly floured surface, use your hands to stretch the pizza dough into a thin

round, about 8 inches. Place it in the prepared pan. Spread the dough with the tomato sauce. Sprinkle with half of the cheese. Arrange the sliced chicken sausage on top, and scatter the pepper over. Sprinkle with the remaining cheese.

6. BAKE until the edges are crisp and lightly browned, and the cheese is melted, about 10 to 12 minutes. Remove from oven, and sprinkle with scallions and basil, if using. Let pizza stand about 2 to 3 minutes before eating.

Cobb Salad

This lunchtime favorite gets a low calorie makeover by using yogurt and buttermilk in place of mayonnaise for a creamy blue cheese dressing. Substitute sliced ham for bacon and cut the calories even more!

SERVES 4
Calories per serving: 471

2	tablespoons fresh lemon juice
$\frac{1}{4}$	cup finely chopped fresh flat-leaf parsley
1	tablespoon olive oil, plus more for oiling grill
$\frac{1}{4}$	teaspoon salt
$\frac{1}{2}$	teaspoon pepper
1	pound chicken breasts, pounded to an even $\frac{1}{3}$-inch thickness
1	ounce crumbled blue cheese (about $\frac{1}{4}$ cup)
$\frac{1}{4}$	cup plain nonfat yogurt
2	tablespoons nonfat or low-fat buttermilk
1	head romaine lettuce, chopped
2	thin slices low-sodium ham, sliced
$\frac{1}{4}$	cup shredded sharp cheddar cheese
2	avocados, seeded, peeled, and cut into $\frac{1}{2}$-inch cubes
2	tomatoes, cut into $\frac{1}{2}$-inch cubes
2	scallions, sliced

1. WHISK together lemon juice, parsley, oil, salt, and $\frac{1}{4}$ teaspoon pepper in a large, shallow dish. Add chicken, turning to coat, and marinate for at least 2 hours and up to overnight.

2. PREHEAT a grill to medium or heat a well-seasoned grill pan over medium heat. Lightly oil grill grate or pan. Grill chicken, turning to create crosshatch marks, until cooked through, about 10 minutes total. Let stand for 10 minutes, then cut into $\frac{1}{2}$ inch cubes.

3. STIR together blue cheese, yogurt, buttermilk, and remaining $\frac{1}{4}$ teaspoon pepper. Pour over lettuce and toss until well coated. Divide lettuce among 4 serving dishes. Divide ham, cheddar cheese, avocados, tomatoes, scallions, and chicken cubes among dishes, arranging each ingredient in a line to create a rainbow of toppings. Serve immediately.

Tip

Yogurt and buttermilk stand in for mayonnaise in the blue cheese dressing.

Sautéed Tequila Lime Shrimp Tacos with Mango and Pineapple Salsa and Spicy Black Beans

Redolent with spices, kissed by chiles, and with a hint of tequila, these shrimp tacos are the perfect bite. Light but satisfying, served with spicy black beans and a mango and pineapple salsa, they make us wish every day was Cinco de Mayo.

SERVES 4

Calories per serving, shrimp tacos: 413
Calories per serving, mango and pineapple salsa: 76
Calories per serving, spicy black beans: 110

For the shrimp tacos:

2   to 4 tablespoons olive oil
1   garlic clove, chopped
½   teaspoon ground cumin
    Pinch red pepper flakes
1   pound medium shrimp, deveined
3   tablespoons high-quality tequila
    Salt, to taste
1   teaspoon dried chipotle powder
2   to 3 tablespoons cilantro, chopped
4   whole wheat tortillas

For the mango and pineapple salsa:

1   large, ripe mango, chopped
¼   cup red onions, chopped
¼   cup red bell pepper, chopped
1   8-ounce can pineapple tidbits
    in juice, drained
1   tablespoon freshly squeezed
    lime juice
1   to 2 tablespoons cilantro, chopped
    Salt, to taste

For the spicy black beans:

2   tablespoons olive oil
2   tablespoons onion, chopped
1   garlic clove, chopped
1   tablespoon ground cumin
1   14-ounce can black beans
2   tablespoons red pepper flakes

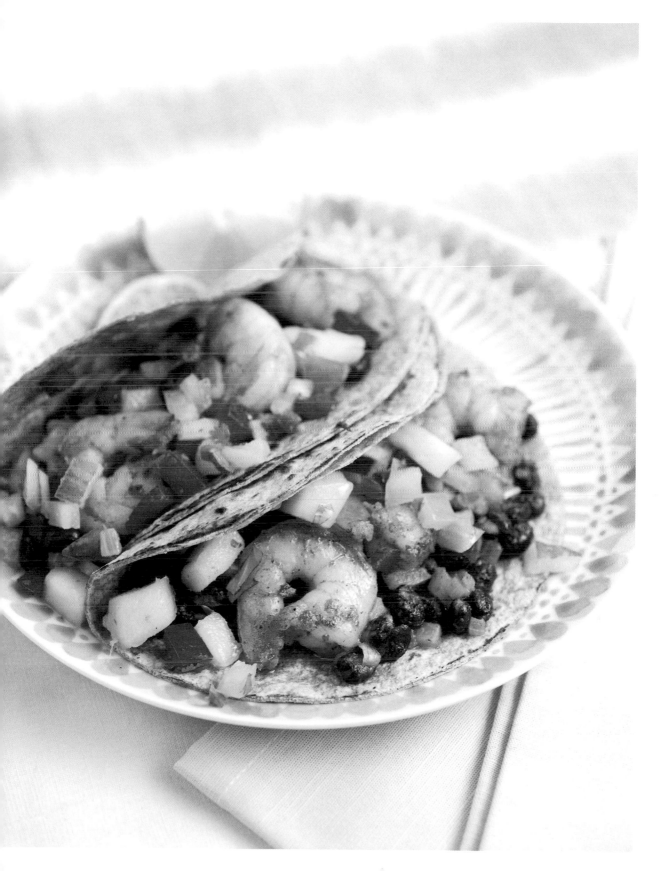

1. TO MAKE THE SHRIMP TACOS: In a large skillet over medium heat, add the olive oil. Add the chopped garlic and cook for about 1 minute. Add the cumin and red pepper flakes and let the flavors blend together. Add the shrimp and toss. Carefully add the tequila and flambé. Season with salt and add the dried chipotle powder. Once shrimp are cooked, add the chopped cilantro and toss.

2. IN A SEPARATE NONSTICK SKILLET over low heat, heat a whole wheat tortilla until pliable, about 2 minutes on each side.

3. PLACE one tortilla per person and serve three shrimp in each taco.

4. TO MAKE THE SPICY BLACK BEANS: In a saucepan over medium heat, add the olive oil, chopped onion, and chopped garlic clove. Sweat the onions for about 2 minutes. Add the cumin and the black beans. Stir and add the red pepper flakes. Simmer for about 5 minutes.

5. TO MAKE THE MANGO AND PINEAPPLE SALSA: Peel the mango and chop into small dice and place in a bowl. Chop the yellow and red bell peppers and add to the bowl with the mango. Add the drained pineapple tidbits and chopped red onion and toss together. Squeeze some lime juice over and toss. Add the chopped cilantro, salt to taste, and toss. Refrigerate until ready to serve.

Mango-Glazed Salmon with Spinach Salad

We love salmon because it's easy and always hits the spot, especially with this Asian-accented mango glaze. It's just perfect sitting atop a spinach salad freshened up with pear, bean sprouts, and toasted sliced almonds.

SERVES 2
Calories per serving: 478

For the salmon:
2 tablespoons soy sauce
1 teaspoon minced ginger
1 (3-inch) cinnamon stick
1 teaspoon rice vinegar
5 ounces mango nectar
2 (6-ounce) salmon fillets, about 1-inch thick

For the dressing:
3 tablespoons rice vinegar
1 tablespoon sesame oil
1 teaspoon ginger (fresh grated)
1 tablespoon orange juice

For the spinach salad:
1 bunch fresh spinach
1 thinly sliced Bosc pear
   Shredded carrots
   Asian bean sprouts
2 tablespoons toasted sliced almonds (optional)

1. TO MAKE THE SALMON: Stir together first 5 ingredients in a small saucepan. Bring to a boil; reduce heat, and simmer, uncovered, 15 minutes or until reduced by half. Pour mango mixture through a wire-mesh strainer; discard solids. Return mango mixture to saucepan; keep warm.

2. PLACE salmon on a rack in a broiler pan coated with cooking spray. Broil 5½ inches from heat 5 minutes. Brush fish with ½ mango mixture. Broil 3 more minutes or until fish flakes with a fork. Spoon remaining mango glaze evenly over fish.

3. TO MAKE THE SPINACH SALAD: Chop the spinach rough cut, thinly slice the Bosc pear into strips, shred the carrots on a grater, add bean sprouts, toss in sliced almonds if desired. Lightly toss the ingredients all together in a mixing bowl with the dressing.

Steak with Cauliflower "Mash" Potatoes

The flat iron steak—today's hippest cut of meat—is also one of the leanest, most flavorful and affordable steaks around. Rubbed with fragrant rosemary and served alongside cauliflower mashed potatoes, it's a steakhouse adventure that's as easy on the waist as it is on the expense account.

SERVES 4
Calories per serving: 389

For the rosemary salt:

2   tablespoons chopped fresh rosemary (from about 4 medium sprigs)
2   tablespoons coarse salt
½   teaspoon coarsely ground black pepper

For the cauliflower mashed potatoes:

½   large head cauliflower, broken into florets (about 8 cups)
½   cup nonfat buttermilk
1   pound Yukon Gold potatoes, peeled, quartered lengthwise, and sliced ½ inch thick
     Salt
½–¾ cup low-fat milk
     Pepper
1   tablespoon butter
2   scallions, chopped

For the steak:

1   pound lean steak, preferably flank, about 1¼ inches thick
1   tablespoon balsamic vinegar
8   cups shredded romaine lettuce
1½   cups halved cherry tomatoes
¼   cup chopped fresh mint

1. FOR THE ROSEMARY SALT, combine chopped rosemary and salt on a cutting board and chop together. Stir in the pepper; transfer to a small bowl, and set aside.

2. FOR THE CAULIFLOWER MASHED POTATOES, place the cauliflower in a steamer basket, set over boiling water, cover, and steam 15 minutes. Transfer to a food processor, add the buttermilk and ¼ cup of the milk, and puree until very smooth, about 2 minutes. Meanwhile, place potatoes in a saucepan, add cold salted water to cover by about 2 inches, bring to a boil, reduce heat, and simmer until tender, about 15 minutes. Drain,

return to the saucepan, and heat over medium heat for 1 to 2 minutes to dry. Mash with a potato masher. Add the cauliflower puree, $\frac{1}{4}$ cup milk, 1 teaspoon salt, and $\frac{1}{4}$ teaspoon pepper. Stir to blend, and heat over medium-low heat, adding more milk as needed for a creamy consistency. Stir in the butter and the scallions. Cover, and set aside to keep warm.

3. HEAT a grill or grill pan. Sprinkle the steak on both sides generously with the rosemary salt, pressing it into the meat. (Reserve the remainder for another use.) Grill the steak 4 minutes on one side. Turn, and grill to rare, 3 to 4 more minutes. Remove to a plate and let stand 5 minutes. Thinly slice the beef against the grain. Add the vinegar to the pan and stir to incorporate any pan juices.

4. TO SERVE, make a bed of lettuce on each of four plates. Arrange one-quarter of the steak slices on top of the lettuce. Spoon on some of the cauliflower mashed potatoes. Scatter tomatoes over all, drizzle with the balsamic-meat juices, and garnish with the chopped mint.

Tips

1. A flank steak is a relatively lean, inexpensive, but exquisitely flavorful and tender cut of beef, more and more readily available at supermarkets.

....

2. An herb salt is a fast and easy way to add flavor to meats and vegetables. Store leftover herb salt at room temperature, and use on poultry, fish, other meats, or roasted vegetables.

....

3. This low-calorie version of mashed potatoes replaces some of the potato with cauliflower, and milk or cream with a combination of buttermilk and low-fat milk. Butter can be replaced by olive oil.

....

4. Balsamic vinegar is useful in low-fat cooking because it adds a lot of flavor, without a lot of acidity – the net result is a sweet-and-sour taste. Whisked with the meat juices here, it makes an instant, nonfat sauce; the beef juices balance the acidity of the vinegar.

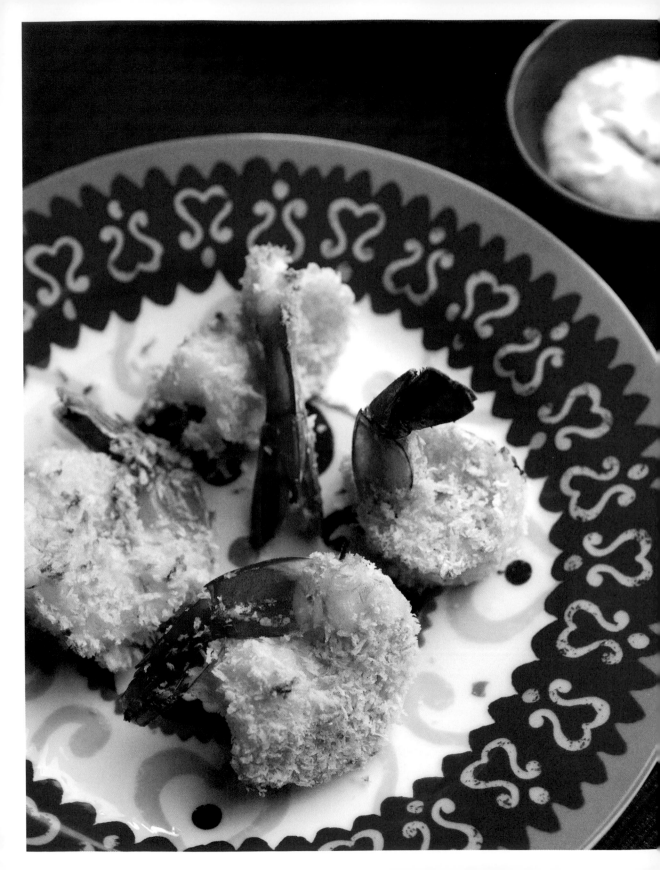

Breaded Not Fried Panko-Crusted Shrimp

Panko crumbs are the best way to get beautifully crisp shrimp in this delightful dish. Mustard and dill add a Nordic touch, while a hint of heat ties these flavors up in a beautiful bundle.

SERVES 4
Calories per serving: 289

2	tablespoons mayonnaise
2	tablespoons creamy dill mustard
2	tablespoons capers, drained and chopped
2	egg whites
½	teaspoon salt
2	cups Panko crumbs
¼	teaspoon cayenne pepper
1	pound jumbo shrimp, peeled, deveined, and butterflied

1. STIR together mayonnaise, mustard, and capers in a small bowl for dipping sauce; set aside.

2. PREHEAT oven to 475 degrees. Whisk egg whites with ¼ teaspoon salt in a shallow dish until frothy. Toss together crumbs, cayenne, and remaining ¼ teaspoon salt in a shallow dish. Dip each shrimp in egg whites, dredge in panko crumbs, and place on a rimmed baking sheet. Bake until shrimp cooks through and crumbs are golden, about 12 minutes.

3. SERVE hot with the dipping sauce.

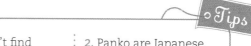

°Tips

1. If you can't find creamy dill mustard, combine 1½ tablespoons Dijon mustard with 1 teaspoon fresh lemon juice and 2 teaspoons finely chopped fresh dill.

2. Panko are Japanese breadcrumbs that are light and crunchy. Look for them online or in the ethnic aisle of your supermarket.

Sautéed Spinach with Grilled Turkey Sausage and Red Pepper and Rosemary Corn Bread

Lemon juice and lemon zest really bring out the fresh flavors in this easy sauté. Serve it with this simple yet satisfying red pepper and rosemary corn bread and feed your soul.

SERVES 4
Calories per serving, sausage and spinach sauté: 272
Calories per serving, red pepper and rosemary corn bread: 168

For the sausage and spinach sauté:
1   tablespoon olive oil
1   pound lean turkey sausage, about 1 package sliced into 1-inch rounds
2   cloves garlic, minced
3   10-ounce packages organic baby spinach
1   lemon
$\frac{1}{4}$ cup chicken broth, low sodium
1   teaspoon salt
$\frac{1}{4}$ teaspoon pepper

For the red pepper and rosemary corn bread:
1   whole red pepper
$\frac{1}{2}$ cup self-rising flour (or see substitute box)
1   cup fine polenta (cornmeal)
$\frac{1}{2}$ teaspoon baking soda
$\frac{1}{4}$ teaspoon salt
$1\frac{1}{2}$ teaspoons dry or fresh rosemary leaves, chopped very fine
$\frac{1}{4}$ cup of pitted black olives (optional)
2   medium free-range eggs
1   cup buttermilk
1   tablespoon honey

> **Self-rising flour substitute:**
> Substitute 1 cup all-purpose flour, $1\frac{1}{2}$ teaspoons baking powder and $\frac{1}{2}$ teaspoon salt for each cup of self-rising flour

1. PREHEAT the oven to 350 degrees for the red pepper and rosemary corn bread.

2. TO MAKE THE SAUSAGE AND SPINACH: Heat a Dutch oven over medium heat; add the oil and sauté the sliced sausage and garlic. Zest the lemon and set aside. Juice the lemon and set aside. Add spinach, lemon juice and zest, and chicken stock, cover and cook until spinach is

cooked down, about 5 minutes. Halfway through cooking toss spinach mixture with tongs. Season with salt and pepper.

3. TO MAKE THE RED PEPPER AND ROSEMARY CORN BREAD: Heat the loaf pan in the oven while the oven is warming up and you are preparing the recipe.

4. PUT the red pepper (halved and middle removed) onto a baking sheet. Place under a hot grill, skin side up, for 10 minutes until the skin is blistered and blackened.

5. REMOVE the red pepper from the oven and immediately place it into a small plastic bag and steam for a further 5 minutes. Carefully peel the skin from the red pepper. Slice thinly.

6. COMBINE the self-rising flour, cornmeal, baking soda, salt, and rosemary in a large mixing bowl. Set aside.

7. IN ANOTHER SMALLER BOWL, whisk the eggs, buttermilk, and honey with a fork until well combined. Add the red peppers. Mix into the dry ingredients, trying to avoid breaking up the peppers as much as possible. If you decide to add the pitted olives to the corn bread, now's the time. Just dice them up and add with the dry ingredients.

8. TAKE the hot pan out of the oven and brush over a little olive oil. Sprinkle with a little cornmeal all over and add in the bread mixture. This will prevent the bread from sticking to the base and sides.

9. BAKE in the middle of the oven at 350 degrees for 35 to 45 minutes or until a skewer inserted into the bread comes out clean.

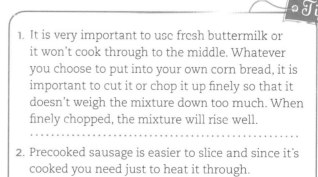

Tips

1. It is very important to use fresh buttermilk or it won't cook through to the middle. Whatever you choose to put into your own corn bread, it is important to cut it or chop it up finely so that it doesn't weigh the mixture down too much. When finely chopped, the mixture will rise well.

2. Precooked sausage is easier to slice and since it's cooked you need just to heat it through.

3. Try boosting flavor with ⅓ cup frozen or fresh cooked corn.

Skinny Down-Home Chicken Pot Pie

Premade phyllo dough makes the scary part of assembling pot pie a breeze, and leaves you plenty of time to get the chicken and veggies just the way you like them for this quintessential hearty comfort food.

SERVES 6
Calories per serving: 372

3	tablespoons olive oil
¼	cup all-purpose flour
1	small onion, diced (about 1.5 ounces)
2	garlic cloves, minced
1	leek, chopped (about 1 ounce)
1	large carrot, chopped (about 1 ounce)
1	celery stalk (about 1 ounce)
2	red potatoes, skin on, diced (about 6 ounces)
2	turnips, peeled and diced (about 4 ounces)
2	boneless, skinless chicken breasts, cut into small cubes
2	boneless, skinless chicken thighs, cut into small cubes
1	bay leaf
2	sprigs of fresh thyme
1	tablespoon salt
1	teaspoon freshly ground pepper
2½	cups chicken stock
6	sheets of phyllo dough
1	tablespoon olive oil, for brushing
1	9-by-9-inch cake pan

1. PREHEAT the oven to 350 degrees. Thaw 6 sheets of phyllo dough overnight in the refrigerator or one hour before using. Bring the chicken stock to a simmer and keep warm.

2. IN A 6-QUART POT, add the olive oil and flour and cook until lightly golden, about 3 minutes. Add the onion, garlic, leek, carrot, celery, red potato, and turnips and stir with a wooden spoon, making sure the bottom does not get too dry. Add the chicken, bay leaf, and sprigs of thyme and continue stirring for about 3 minutes, so that everything is coated with the flour mixture.

3. ADD the warm chicken stock, stir and scrape the bottom of the pot to get all the color into the mixture and keep it from scorching. Bring to a boil then lower to a simmer. Let the mixture simmer, covered, for another 5 to 7 minutes until it becomes thick and the chicken is opaque. Remove from heat and reserve.

4. MEANWHILE, take 6 sheets of phyllo dough and, with a knife, cut out a square slightly larger than the rim of the 9-by-9-inch cake pan and brush with some olive oil. Set aside.

5. REMOVE the bay leaf and thyme sprigs from the chicken mixture and transfer the chicken to the cake pan. Top with the phyllo dough and press it down firmly with your hands. Place the pie on a baking sheet and bake in the oven at 350 degrees for 30 minutes, turning the tray around halfway through the cooking time. Remove from the oven, let cool for 10 minutes, cut into six portions and serve.

Mediterranean Chicken

This boldly flavored Italian sauce is so simple to make and it'll dress up salmon, steak, or in this case, grilled, butterflied chicken breasts. The juicy, herbaceous salsa verde leaves you with a beautiful plate, bursting with exciting and dynamic flavors.

SERVES 4
Calories per serving: 370

For the Chicken:
2   tablespoons extra virgin olive oil
1   lemon, washed and quartered
3   cloves garlic, peeled and smashed
1   teaspoon salt
1/4 teaspoon freshly ground pepper
3   branches fresh rosemary, or
     1 teaspoon dried
4   boneless, skinless chicken breasts,
     butterflied

For the side of tomatoes:
1   tablespoon olive oil
1   garlic clove, whole
1   pint cherry tomatoes
     Splash of balsamic vinegar

For the Salsa Verde:
1   cup flat leaf parsley, chopped
1   cup mint leaves, chopped
2   cups basil, chopped
1/3 cup extra-virgin olive oil
3   garlic cloves, finely chopped
3   tablespoons capers, rinsed
     and chopped
4   anchovy fillets, bones removed,
     soaked and chopped
1   tablespoon Dijon mustard
1   tablespoon red wine vinegar
1/8 teaspoon freshly ground pepper,
     or more to taste
     Coarse sea salt, to taste

1. TO MARINATE THE CHICKEN: In a large plastic sealable bag, squeeze the juice from the lemon and add the lemon. Add all the remaining ingredients, seal carefully, and massage the marinade into the chicken. Refrigerate for 30 minutes, or even overnight.

2. TO MAKE THE SALSA VERDE: Mix all ingredients in a small bowl. Set aside until serving. Refrigerate if made earlier in the day and remove an hour or so before serving.

3. TO COOK THE CHICKEN: Lightly spray a stovetop cast iron griddle with oil and heat over medium high heat until smoking.

4. REMOVE the chicken from the marinade and pat off excess marinade. Place the chicken on the griddle and cook about 2 to 3 minutes per side. Turn the chicken and cook 2 more minutes, until cooked through.

5. TO MAKE THE TOMATOES: Heat the oil in a small sauté pan over medium high heat. Add the garlic and tomatoes and splash of balsamic vinegar and sauté for 2-3 minutes, until the tomatoes are warmed through. Crush lightly with a wooden spoon and serve.

6. PLACE the chicken on a platter and top with the salsa verde with the tomatoes on the side.

Tips

1. Grilled, butterflied chicken breasts—the butterfly technique is so simple and your eye sees a bountiful and beautiful plate.

2. You can freeze the chicken in the marinade as well.

3. You can pulse the whole herbs and all the salsa verde ingredients in a small food processor rather than chopping herbs by hand. Take care not to finely puree, as the mixture should be slightly coarse.

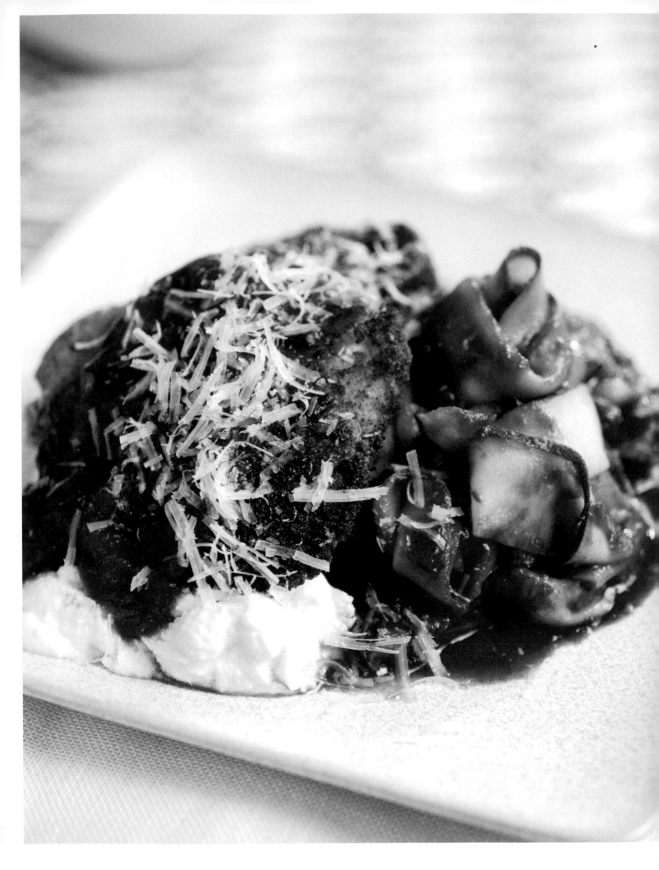

Cheezy Chicken Parmesan with Zucchini "Pasta"

Zucchini sliced paper-thin stands in for pappardelle pasta and low-fat ricotta brings the creamy feel of a high-fat pasta dish. Wheat bread-crumbs and a quick dip in light oil give a delectable crunch to the chicken cutlets.

SERVES 4
Calories per serving: 350

For the tomato sauce and zucchini pappardelle:

- 2 tablespoons olive oil, divided
- ¼ red onion, coarsely chopped
- 3 cloves garlic, sliced thin
  Salt
- 1 (28-ounce) can peeled plum tomatoes, preferably San Marzano, in juice, mashed
- 1 sprig fresh basil
  Pepper
- ¼ cup fresh parsley leaves, chopped
- 4 zucchini (about 1½ pounds), trimmed at both ends

For the chicken:

- ¼ cup freshly grated Parmesan cheese, plus 2 tablespoons extra, for serving
- ¼ cup dried whole wheat or white breadcrumbs
- 1 large egg white, lightly beaten with a fork
- 1 pound boneless, skinless chicken breasts, split in half to make 6 to 8 large, thin cutlets
  Pepper
- 4 teaspoons olive oil, plus 2 teaspoons extra for serving
- ¼ cup part-skim ricotta cheese

1. FOR THE SAUCE, heat 1 tablespoon of the oil in a large skillet over medium-low heat. Add the onion, garlic, and ½ teaspoon salt. Cook, stirring, 1 minute. Cover, reduce heat to very low and cook until vegetables are softened, about 5 minutes. (Check a few times during cooking; if vegetables begin to brown, add 2 teaspoons water and stir.) Add the tomatoes with juice, basil, and another ½ teaspoon salt. Bring to a simmer, cover and simmer gently 5 minutes. Then simmer very gently, partially cov-ered, until thickened, about 20 minutes. Season with ⅛ teaspoon pepper.

2. MEANWHILE, using a mandolin or vegetable peeler, slice the zucchini lengthwise into ⅛-inch-thick long pappardelle-like strips, turning the zucchini and slicing on 4 sides only until you see the center seeds. Discard the centers.

3. REMOVE the tomato sauce to a bowl with a rubber spatula; no need to clean the skillet. Heat the remaining 1 tablespoon of oil in the skillet over medium heat. Add the zucchini and ¼ teaspoon salt. Cover and cook until wilted, tossing often with tongs for even cooking, 8 to 10 minutes. Return the tomato sauce to the pan, add 1 tablespoon of the parsley, and season with ⅛ teaspoon pepper; cover and set aside.

4. ON A PLATE, combine the breadcrumbs, ¼ cup grated Parmesan, and the remaining chopped parsley. Place the egg white on a second plate. Sprinkle chicken on both sides with salt and pepper. Dip the chicken into the egg whites, and then into the breadcrumb mixture to coat completely; set aside on a large plate or platter.

5. HEAT 2 teaspoons oil in each of two nonstick 10-inch skillets over medium-high heat. Add half of the chicken to each skillet and cook until lightly browned on one side, 2 to 3 minutes. Flip, and cook until chicken is firm, and lightly browned on the other side, 1 to 3 more minutes.

6. TO SERVE, rewarm the zucchini in the tomato sauce over medium heat. Use tongs to make a "twist" of zucchini pappardelle on each of 4 plates. Lean chicken cutlets against the side of zucchini. Scoop 1 tablespoon ricotta onto each plate, and spoon remaining tomato sauce on top of the chicken. To garnish each plate, drizzle chicken with ½ teaspoon olive oil, and sprinkle with 1 teaspoon Parmesan.

Tips

1. This recipe uses a minimum of Parmesan cheese in the breading, and very little oil for sautéing, so that you can add a little extra of both on top of the finished dish—where you can taste it quite directly—for an additional kick of bright flavor.

2. One pound of chicken tenders may be substituted for chicken breasts.

3. Zucchini sliced thin on an inexpensive mandolin or v-slicer makes a low-fat, low-calorie substitute for pasta.

Spaghetti Carbonara

Simple, classic, and oh-so Italian, carbonara is what spaghetti was born to become. Al dente pasta paired with salty smoky bacon, peas, and Parmesan is a culinary revelation—perfect and easy. Too bad life can't be like this more often.

SERVES 4
Calories per serving: 412

For the spaghetti:

3   slices bacon
1   teaspoon olive oil
1   small onion, diced
$\frac{1}{3}$ cup low-fat (1%) milk
1   large egg
8   ounces spaghetti
1   cup frozen peas
1$\frac{1}{2}$ ounces Parmesan cheese, finely grated (6 tablespoons)
$\frac{1}{4}$ cup sliced fresh flat-leaf parsley
    Salt, to taste
    Pepper, to taste

1. COOK the bacon in a large skillet over medium heat, turning occasionally until browned and crisp, about 6 minutes. Drain pan and dry bacon on paper towels; keep the skillet on the heat. Add the oil and onion and cook, stirring occasionally, until softened and translucent, about 3 minutes. Remove from the heat. Whisk together the milk and egg in a large serving bowl until well-combined. Stir in the onion.

2. BRING a large saucepan of salted water to a boil. Add spaghetti, and cook according to the directions on the package. Two minutes before the spaghetti is done, stir in the peas. Drain and immediately transfer to the milk mixture. Toss until the pasta is well-coated. Add the cheese, parsley, $\frac{1}{2}$ teaspoon salt, and $\frac{1}{4}$ teaspoon pepper and toss well. Crumble the bacon into small pieces over the spaghetti, and toss. Serve immediately.

Tip

This is best with regular pasta; whole wheat, or whole grain pasta competes with the taste of the sauce.

Supreme Quesadilla with Poblano Peppers

Mexicans have known that freshness and a little spice go a long way toward eating healthy, as proved by this earthy roasted pepper quesadilla. Lime and onion give the guacamole depth without compromise. Corn tortillas are naturally lower in fat and calories than bread but every bit as satisfying.

SERVES 4
Calories per serving: 272

For the quesadillas:
1   poblano chile
1   teaspoon vegetable oil
1   large white onion
$\frac{1}{4}$ teaspoon salt
    Freshly ground black pepper,
    to taste
8   corn tortillas
4   ounces shredded low-fat
    cheddar cheese

For the guacamole:
1   Hass avocado
$\frac{1}{2}$ large tomato, cored and diced
$\frac{1}{2}$ tablespoon fresh lime juice
$\frac{1}{4}$ teaspoon salt

To serve:
$\frac{1}{4}$ cup reduced-fat sour cream

1. ROAST the poblano chile over an open flame with a burner on using a pair of tongs to hold over the fire. Turn the chile occasionally and roast until completely blackened. Alternatively, broil on a baking sheet, turning, until blackened. Transfer to a bowl and cover with plastic wrap and let stand for 10 to 15 minutes.

2. WHILE THE CHILE COOLS, make the guacamole. Seed, peel, and dice the avocado and transfer to a bowl along with the diced tomato, lime juice, and salt. Stir and mash with a fork or spoon until well combined and set aside.

3. PEEL, stem and seed the cooled poblano chile and cut it crosswise into thin strips. Heat the oil in a large skillet over medium heat. Add the onion and poblano chile strips and season with $\frac{1}{4}$ teaspoon of salt and freshly ground pepper, stirring occasionally. Add about 2 tablespoons of water if the mixture becomes too dry. Cover with a lid and cook until the onions are softened and translucent, about 9 minutes. Remove from heat and reserve warm.

4. HEAT a separate skillet over low to medium heat. Place 2 tortillas and warm them, turning occasionally, until pliable, about 2-3 minutes. Remove one tortilla and reserve. Sprinkle a thin, even layer of cheese on a tortilla in the skillet. Top with an even layer of the warm chile and onion mixture, then another thin layer of cheese. Center the reserved warm tortilla over the cheese and heat until the bottom tortilla is browned in spots, about 1 minute. Carefully flip quesadilla and cook until the other side is brown and the cheese is completely melted, about 2 minutes. Place on a baking sheet and keep warm in the oven. Repeat with the remaining tortillas and filling.

5. CUT each quesadilla in quarters and serve with the guacamole and sour cream.

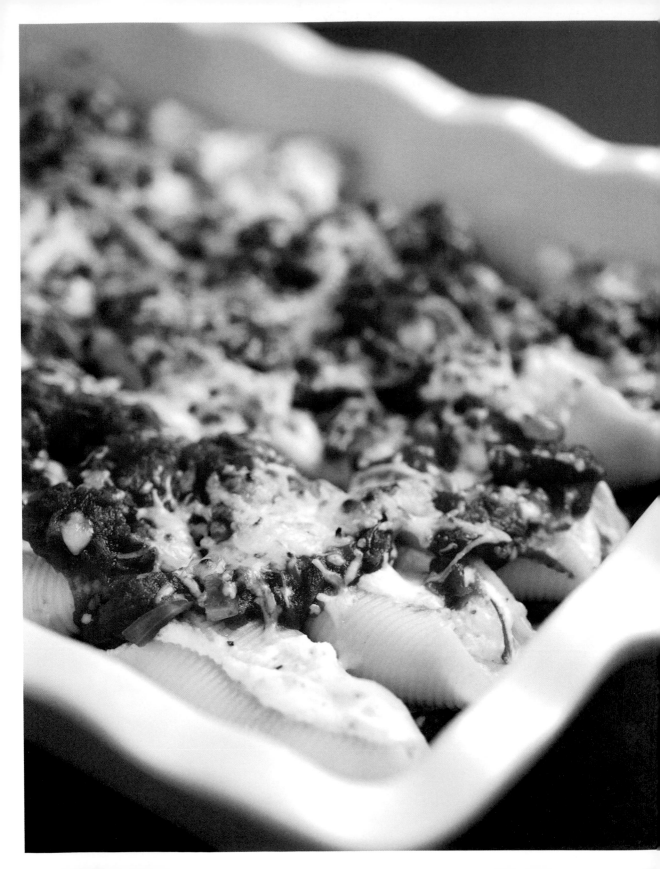

Stuffed Shells

It's important to remember that zucchini is your friend. It's a real chameleon in the kitchen, taking the place of noodles or in this case cheese, adding weight to the dish, not to you.

SERVES 10
Calories per serving: 331

12 ounces (1 box) jumbo pasta shells (approximately 40 shells)

For the tomato sauce:
1 (28-ounce) can peeled plum tomatoes in juice
1 (14-ounce) can peeled plum tomatoes in juice
2 teaspoons olive oil
$3/4$ cup roughly chopped red onion
4 cloves garlic, sliced thin
  Salt
2 sprigs fresh basil
  Pepper

For the stuffing:
  1-pound bag baby spinach
  Salt and pepper
2 teaspoons olive oil, plus extra for serving
2 medium zucchini, halved lengthwise, and sliced thin
2 scallions, chopped
2 cups (16 ounces) part-skim ricotta cheese
$1\frac{1}{2}$ cups shredded reduced-fat, part-skim mozzarella cheese
1 thin slice ham, chopped
2 tablespoons chopped parsley
$1/2$ cup grated Parmesan cheese
  Pinch grated nutmeg

1. SPRAY a baking sheet lightly with cooking spray. Bring a large pot of salted water to a boil. Add the shells, and partially cook—they should have started to become tender but will still be firm to the bite, 6 to 7 minutes. Drain in a colander, and immediately transfer to the oiled baking sheet, spreading them out in a single layer so that they don't stick together. Let cool.

2. FOR THE SAUCE, pour the tomatoes into a bowl and mash with your hands, or pulse in food processor to chop. Heat the oil in a large saucepan over medium-low heat. Add the onion and garlic. Cook, stirring, for 1 minute. Cover, reduce heat to very low and cook until vegetables are softened, about 5 minutes. (Check a few times during cooking; if vegetables begin to brown, add 2 teaspoons water and stir.) Add the tomatoes with juice, basil, and $1/2$ teaspoon salt. Bring to a simmer, cover, and simmer gently 5 minutes. Then simmer very gently, partially covered, until thickened, about 20 minutes. Season with $1/8$ teaspoon pepper. Scrape into another container with a rubber spatula; set aside.

3. ADD the spinach and $\frac{1}{2}$ teaspoon salt to the skillet. Place over medium heat, cover and cook, tossing every now and then with tongs for even cooking, until wilted, 5 to 6 minutes. Drain, and let cool, then squeeze out as much liquid as you can, and chop. Transfer to a bowl; set aside.

4. IN THE SAME SKILLET, heat the oil over medium heat. Add the zucchini and $\frac{1}{4}$ teaspoon salt and cook, stirring every now and then, until tender and lightly browned, 5 to 7 minutes. Add scallions during the final 1 minute. Add to the bowl with the spinach. Add the ricotta, the ham, $\frac{1}{2}$ cup of the mozzarella, the parsley, $\frac{1}{8}$ teaspoon pepper, and the nutmeg, and stir to combine.

5. PREHEAT the oven to 350 degrees.

6. SPOON a thin layer of sauce over the bottom of two 9-by-13-inch baking dishes. Fill the cooked shells with the cheese mixture, about 1 tablespoon per shell, and arrange the shells side by side in a single layer in the pre-pared dishes. Spoon the remaining sauce over the shells, then sprinkle each with $\frac{1}{2}$ cup of the mozzarella, and $\frac{1}{4}$ cup of the Parmesan.

7. COVER with aluminum foil and bake until the filling is heated through and the cheese is melted, 25 to 30 minutes.

Tip

Cooked zucchini stands in for some of the cheese in the traditional ricotta filling, adding bulk and moisture. Other vegetables can be substituted, including sautéed mushrooms, or baked butternut squash.

Eggplant Stacks

Let smoky grilled eggplant stamp your tastebuds' passport for a flavor trip to the Greek Isles. Feta, tomatoes, and pesto join eggplant in this delicious layered construction that stacks up favorably against fattier moussaka or lasagna.

SERVES 4
Calories per serving, 2 stacks per person: 596

4   eggplants, thinly sliced rounds, about 2 pounds
4   tablespoons extra-virgin olive oil
4   tablespoons balsamic vinegar
1   lemon, juiced
1¼ cups store-bought pesto
4   to 5 tomatoes, thinly sliced
1¼ cups feta, crumbled
½   cup basil
    Salt and pepper

1. LAY the eggplant slices on a sheet pan, lightly sprinkle with salt and pepper.

2. MIX together the olive oil, balsamic vinegar, and lemon juice, and lightly brush the eggplant slices.

3. HEAT the broiler or grill pan, or low gas grill. Grill or broil the eggplant, turning over occasionally, until eggplant is very tender, 6 to 10 minutes, do not let them burn. Cook low and slow for sweetness. Remove and reserve.

4. PREHEAT oven to 350 degrees.

5. ON BAKING PAN, arrange 4 of the largest eggplant rounds side by side and spread each with thin layer of pesto, then top each with largest tomato rounds. Season tomatoes with salt and pepper and top each with about 1 tablespoon feta and a pinch of chopped basil. Continue to layer, ending with cheese.

6. BAKE in the oven (or on the grill) until cheese begins to melt, about 3-4 minutes. Garnish with fresh lemons.

> **Tip**
>
> If your kids don't like pesto or feta, you can change it up with tomato sauce and mozzarella.

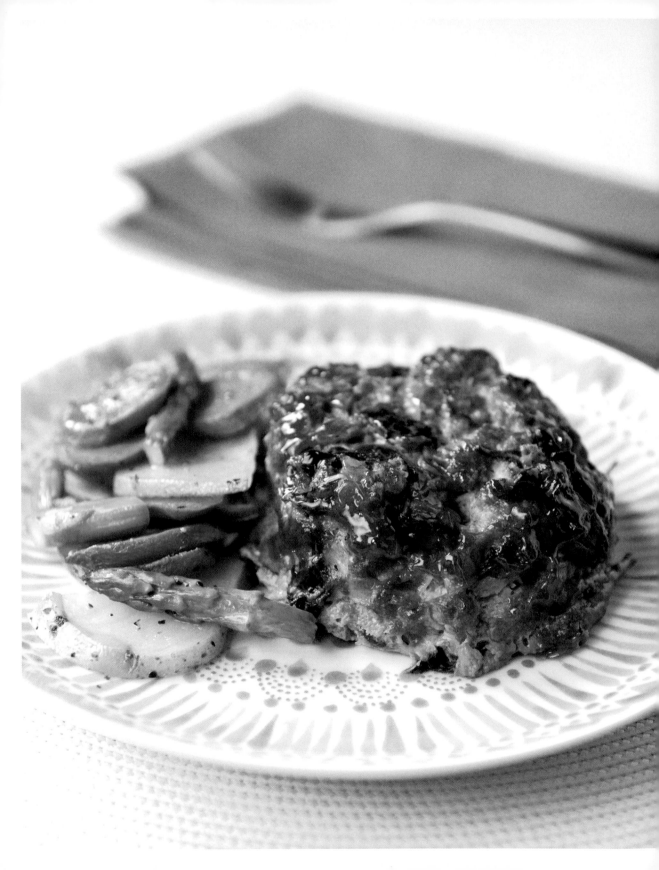

Turkey Mini-Meatloaves with Roasted Root Veggies

Ground turkey is one of those things we really can't live without. It's as versatile as ground beef with so much less of everything bad. Baking the meatloaves in individual portions helps maintain portion control.

SERVES 4
Calories per serving, meatloaves: 227
Calories per serving, roasted root veggies: 121

For the meatloaf:
1   slice whole wheat bread
½   cup skim milk
1   tablespoon plus 1 teaspoon olive oil
1   onion, diced
    5-ounce bag baby spinach leaves
1¼ pounds ground turkey
2   tablespoons finely grated Parmesan
1   large egg
½   teaspoon salt
¼   teaspoon freshly ground black pepper
⅛   teaspoon freshly grated nutmeg

For the glaze:
3   tablespoons ketchup
2   teaspoons Worcestershire sauce
1   teaspoon hot sauce

For the roasted root veggies:
3   large carrots, cut on the bias
2   Yukon Gold potatoes, cut on the bias
¼   cup asparagus (about 4 stalks)
1   teaspoon chopped parsley
1   teaspoon chopped chives
1½ tablespoons olive oil
1   teaspoon salt
¼   teaspoon pepper

1. PREHEAT oven to 375 degrees. Arrange oven racks to accommodate two dishes being cooked simultaneously.

2. GRIND the bread in a food processor until fine crumbs form. Transfer to a large bowl, and pour milk over crumbs.

3. HEAT 1 teaspoon oil in a large skillet, preferably nonstick, over medium heat. Add onion and cook, stirring occasionally, until softened and golden, about 5 minutes. Add spinach, and stir until just wilted, about 30 seconds. Transfer to bowl with soaked crumbs. Add the turkey, cheese, egg, salt, pepper, and nutmeg. Combine the mixture with your hands until well mixed; it will be quite wet.

4. PACK 1 cup of the mixture into a 1-cup dry measuring cup. Invert the

cup onto a rimmed baking sheet, gently shaking the cup to release the mixture. Gently pat the mound to smooth its shape. Repeat with remaining mixture. Bake mini meatloaves until cooked through and golden, about 40 minutes.

5. WHILE THE MEATLOAVES ARE COOKING, make the glaze: In a small bowl combine the ketchup, Worcestershire sauce, and hot sauce. Brush over meatloaves.

6. TO MAKE THE ROASTED ROOT VEGETABLES: On a baking sheet, toss all the vegetables in the olive oil, season with salt and pepper. Add to the oven along with the meatloaf and roast for 30–35 minutes, stirring midway through baking. Remove from the oven and sprinkle with fresh herbs.

Tip

Ground turkey stands in for ground beef; spinach keeps the mixture moist, without adding fat.

Mac and Cheese

Comfort food that doesn't require sweatpants. Everyone's favorite mac and cheese keeps us in form-flattering jeans thanks to multi-grain pasta and smarter cheese choices. So easy to make too.

SERVES 4
Calories per serving: 517

2   cups multi-grain elbow macaroni
1½ tablespoons unsalted butter
2   tablespoons all-purpose flour
1½ cups skim milk, warmed for 1 minute in the microwave, or heated on stove
8   ounces low-fat sharp cheddar cheese, shredded (about 2¼ cups)
2   teaspoons Worcestershire sauce
    Pinch of pepper
    Pinch of freshly grated nutmeg
¼   cup Panko crumbs or whole wheat breadcrumbs

1. PREHEAT the broiler.

2. BRING a large saucepan of salted water to a boil and cook pasta according to package directions.

3. WHILE THE PASTA IS COOKING, melt the butter in a large saucepan over medium heat. Add the flour and cook, whisking constantly until golden, about 2 minutes. Continue whisking and add the milk in a slow, steady stream. Bring the mixture to a steady simmer, whisking constantly, and whisk until thickened, about 2 minutes.

4. DRAIN the pasta in a colander. Remove the sauce from the heat, add the cheese, and stir until the cheese melts. Immediately add the hot, drained pasta and stir until well-coated. Stir in Worcestershire sauce, ¼ teaspoon salt, a pinch of pepper, and the nutmeg.

5. DIVIDE the mac and cheese among four 6-ounce ovenproof ramekins and sprinkle 1 tablespoon breadcrumbs over each. Broil until crumbs are golden and crisp, 1 to 2 minutes, taking care not to let the top burn. Serve immediately.

Tips

1. To make fresh bread-crumbs, process a slice of whole wheat bread in the food processor.

2. Boost flavor, not calories by mixing in fresh chopped herbs or scallions.

Sweet and Sour Pork Chops

Today's pork is lean, delicious, and a joy to cook with—especially when it ends up in this tangy, fruity Asian-inspired sauce. We love to serve it on nutty brown rice to really bring out the complex flavors.

SERVES 4
Calories per serving, pork chops: 290
Calories per serving, brown rice: 175

For the pork chops:
1   tablespoon dry sherry
¼   teaspoon pepper
2   tablespoons low-sodium soy sauce
1½ teaspoons sugar
1   pound (1-inch-thick) boneless pork loin chops, trimmed of any fat, and cut into 1-inch cubes
2   tablespoons pineapple juice
1   tablespoon ketchup
½   teaspoon white vinegar
3   tablespoons canola oil
1   red onion, peeled, trimmed, and cut into 1-inch cubes
2   red (or 1 red and 1 green) bell peppers, stemmed, seeded, and cut into 1-inch cubes

For the brown rice:
1½ cups brown rice
3   cups chicken stock

1. TO MAKE THE PORK CHOPS: Combine sherry, pepper, 1 tablespoon of the soy sauce, and ½ teaspoon of the sugar in a medium bowl. Add pork and gently toss until well-coated. Let marinate in the refrigerator.

2. STIR together pineapple juice, ketchup, vinegar, the remaining tablespoon of soy sauce, and remaining teaspoon of sugar in a small bowl until well-combined.

3. HEAT 1 tablespoon of the oil in a large, nonstick skillet over medium-high heat until hot but not smoking. Add onion and cook, stirring occasionally, until browned but still a little crisp, about 2 minutes.

Transfer to a large dish. Heat another tablespoon oil in the same skillet over medium-high heat until hot but not smoking. Add peppers and cook, stirring occasionally, until browned but still a little crisp, about 3 minutes. Transfer to the same dish.

4. HEAT remaining tablespoon oil in the same skillet over medium-high heat until hot but not smoking. Add the pork cubes, arranging in a single layer. Cook, undisturbed, until a golden-brown crust forms on the bottom, about $1\frac{1}{2}$ minutes. Turn the cubes over and cook until a golden-brown crust forms on the other side, about $1\frac{1}{2}$ minutes. Return onion and peppers to the pan and toss to combine. Add pineapple juice mixture and cook, stirring, until sauce evenly coats everything and thickens slightly, about 2 minutes. Serve immediately.

5. TO MAKE THE BROWN RICE: In a saucepan, bring the stock to a boil and add the rice. Cover with a lid and let simmer for 20 to 30 minutes. Using a fork, fluff the grains and serve.

> Tip
>
> This serves 4 as a one-dish meal with steamed brown or white rice, or eight as one of many dishes in a larger meal.

Green Chile Chicken Enchiladas

Most of what you need to whip up a tray of these tasty enchiladas you probably already have in your fridge or pantry. Just oven-roast a pair of piquant peppers and the rest practically takes care of itself. And as is the case with most real Mexican, fat isn't really an issue.

SERVES 4
Calories per serving: 456

For the Enchiladas:

2	roasted poblano peppers, peeled
1	bunch of cilantro leaves, washed, stems discarded
1	lime, zested and juiced
2	cloves garlic
3/4	cup chicken broth
1	teaspoon salt
1/4	teaspoon freshly ground black pepper
12	corn tortillas
1	cup canned nonfat refried beans
3	cups of leftover roast chicken, shredded
3/4	cup reduced-fat shredded cheese, such as Mexican-style, Monterey Jack, or cheddar
2	scallions, thinly sliced

For the garnish:

chopped fresh cilantro,
1 lime, cut into wedges

1. PREHEAT oven to 425 degrees.

2. LIGHTLY OIL a 9-by-13-inch baking dish with cooking spray or one teaspoon olive oil. In a food processor or a blender, puree the roasted and peeled peppers, cilantro, garlic, lime zest and juice, chicken stock, salt, and pepper until smooth.

3. SPREAD ⅓ cup of the sauce in the prepared baking dish. Top with an overlapping layer of 6 tortillas. Spread refried beans evenly over the tortillas. Top the beans with the shredded chicken mixture, and add ⅓ of the sauce, followed by the remaining 6 tortillas. Pour the remaining sauce over the tortillas. Cover with foil.

4. BAKE the enchiladas until they begin to bubble on the sides, about 20 minutes. Remove the foil; sprinkle cheese and scallions on top. Continue baking until heated through and the cheese is melted, about 5 minutes more. Top with cilantro and serve with lime wedges.

Tip

Can't find poblanos?
Swap 2 green or red
roasted peppers.
Like it spicier? Toss a
jalapeño in the blender.

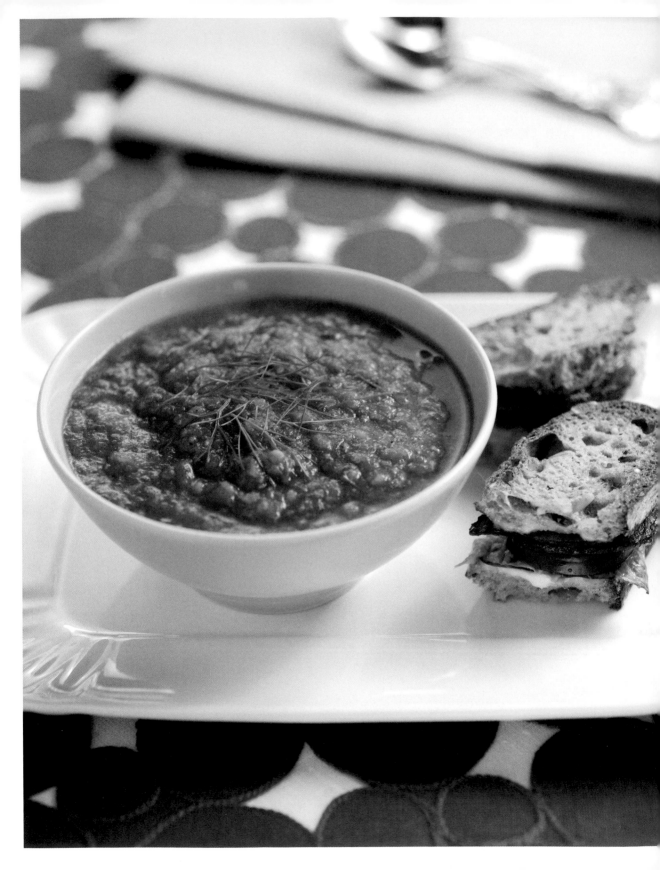

Tomato Fennel Soup and Turkey BLT

Turkey bacon is so tasty in this reworked classic soup and sandwich combo. We like the way a splash of white wine really brightens our tomato soup, and sweet-savory spicing sets these BLTs apart from the ho-hum.

SERVES 4
Calories per serving: 508

For the tomato fennel soup:
2   medium fennel bulbs
2   tablespoons vegetable oil
½   teaspoon salt
¼   teaspoon pepper
4   medium tomatoes, cored and quartered
4   sprigs fresh thyme
½   cup dry white wine
2   teaspoons tomato paste
1   cup low-sodium chicken broth
2   (1-inch-thick) slices whole wheat baguette, toasted
2   teaspoons sugar, if needed

For the sandwiches:
4   slices turkey bacon
1   tablespoon maple syrup
½   teaspoon coarsely ground black pepper
¼   teaspoon cayenne pepper
3   tablespoons mayonnaise
8   (¼-inch-thick) slices whole wheat baguette, lightly toasted
8   leaves iceberg lettuce
1   small tomato, sliced

1. TO MAKE THE SOUP, trim the tops and fronds from the fennel, reserving 8 fronds for garnish. Halve the fennel lengthwise, and remove the cores. Cut the fennel crosswise into ½-inch-thick slices.

2. HEAT the oil in a large saucepan over medium heat. Add the fennel, season with ¼ teaspoon salt and ⅛ teaspoon pepper, and cook, stirring occasionally, until softened and caramelized, about 25 minutes. Add the tomatoes, thyme, and remaining ¼ teaspoon salt and ⅛ teaspoon pepper. Cook, stirring occasionally until the tomatoes break down completely, about 15 minutes. Add the wine, tomato paste, and broth, and simmer 20 minutes. Add the bread and soak it in the soup until completely softened, about 5 minutes.

3. REMOVE the thyme sprigs, transfer soup to a blender or food processor, and blend until completely smooth. Return to the saucepan. (If you prefer

a thinner, smoother soup, strain through a fine-mesh sieve.) Heat over medium-low heat until heated through, about 1 minute. If the tomatoes were not ripe summer fruit, taste and add sugar if needed.

4. WHILE THE SOUP SIMMERS, make the sandwiches: Preheat the oven to 400 degrees. Place the bacon on a baking sheet lined with parchment paper, a nonstick baking mat, or lightly greased foil. Bake until golden, turning once, about 10 minutes. Brush bacon with syrup and sprinkle with both peppers. Bake until golden brown and crisp, about 10 minutes. Break each piece into thirds.

5. SPREAD the mayonnaise on one side of each of the baguette slices. Divide the bacon, lettuce, and tomato among 4 slices of bread. Sandwich with the remaining slices of bread. Serve soup and sandwiches together.

Tips

1. Whole wheat bread can act as a low-fat thickener for all your favorite soups.

2. A stick or immersion blender lets you blend right in the pot for easier clean up.

Portobello Mushroom Tuna Melt

Tuna melt loses the carbs and gets sophisticated yet simple when portobellos are swapped for the usual toast.

SERVES 2
Calories per serving: 539

4   portobello mushrooms, stemmed, gills removed
2   tablespoons olive oil
1   (5-ounce) can albacore tuna packed in water, drained
1   celery stalk, finely chopped
½   cup finely chopped fresh flat-leaf parsley
2   tablespoons fresh lemon juice
    Salt and pepper
4   deli-thin slices Swiss cheese
4   slices tomatoes
½   cup mixed baby greens

1. PREHEAT the broiler. Brush the mushrooms with 1 tablespoon oil. Transfer to a rimmed baking sheet and broil, turning once until softened and cooked through, about 10 minutes.

2. WHILE THE MUSHROOMS ARE COOKING, in a bowl, combine tuna, celery, parsley, lemon juice, ½ teaspoon salt, ¼ teaspoon pepper, and remaining tablespoon oil.

3. REMOVE the mushrooms from the oven. Divide tuna mixture among mushrooms, and spread evenly in caps. Top each with a slice of cheese, and broil until cheese melts, about 2 minutes. Top each mushroom with a tomato slice and 2 tablespoons greens, and serve immediately.

Tip

Try low-fat Swiss instead of regular as a calorie saver. To change up the flavor, try Havarti or cheddar.

Chicken Tetrazzini

Eat creamy chicken tetrazzini without guilt thanks to a little skim milk and whole grain noodles. Roast seasoned white meat chicken for minimum fat and maximum flavor with an unequaled air of indulgence.

SERVES 4
Calories per serving: 450

$3\frac{1}{2}$ tablespoons olive oil
1 pound split, bone-in chicken breasts
1 tablespoon fresh thyme leaves
$\frac{1}{2}$ teaspoon salt
$\frac{1}{4}$ teaspoon pepper
1 pound mushrooms, trimmed and quartered
2 cloves garlic, finely chopped
$1\frac{1}{2}$ tablespoons unsalted butter
1 tablespoon all-purpose flour
$\frac{3}{4}$ cup skim milk, warmed
$\frac{3}{4}$ cup low-sodium chicken stock, warmed
$\frac{1}{4}$ pound whole grain spaghetti
1 cup frozen peas, thawed
2 tablespoons finely grated Parmesan ($\frac{1}{4}$ ounce)

1. PREHEAT oven to 400 degrees. Lightly grease a shallow $1\frac{1}{2}$-quart glass or ceramic baking dish with $\frac{1}{2}$ tablespoon of the oil. Place chicken in the prepared baking dish. Rub with 1 tablespoon oil, sprinkle with thyme leaves, and $\frac{1}{8}$ teaspoon each salt and pepper. Roast until chicken is golden brown, and cooked through, about 25 minutes.

2. MEANWHILE, arrange the mushrooms in a single layer in a 2-quart glass or ceramic baking dish. Add the garlic, $\frac{1}{4}$ teaspoon salt, and the remaining 2 tablespoons oil, and toss to coat. Roast alongside chicken until mushrooms are browned, about 15 minutes.

3. LOWER oven heat to 350 degrees. Set mushrooms aside. When chicken is cool enough to handle, remove skin and bones, and cut meat into $\frac{1}{2}$-inch cubes. Reserve the baking dish.

4. BRING a large saucepan of water to a boil and cook spaghetti according to package directions. Drain in a colander.

5. WHILE THE SPAGHETTI IS COOKING, melt the butter in a large saucepan over medium heat. Add the flour and cook, whisking constantly, until golden, about 2 minutes. Whisking constantly, add the milk, and then the broth in a slow, steady stream. Bring the sauce to a steady simmer, whisking constantly until thickened, about 2 minutes. Season with remaining ⅛ teaspoon each salt and pepper.

6. IN A LARGE BOWL, toss together the spaghetti, peas, mushrooms, and half of the sauce. Transfer to reserved baking dish, making a well in the center. Stir together chicken meat and remaining sauce, and spoon into the well. Sprinkle all over with cheese.

7. BAKE until sauce is bubbling and top is lightly browned, about 15 minutes. Serve immediately.

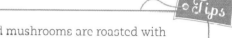

Tips

1. Chicken and mushrooms are roasted with seasonings for richer flavor. Traditional sauces use cream—this one uses a combination of chicken stock and skim milk for a creamy consistency and less fat.

2. Roasting breasts on the bone adds flavor. If you're in a rush, use storebought rotisserie chicken.

Buffalo Chicken Wings

You don't have to give up your fried faves in order to lose weight—you just have to make the recipes work for you. Our roasted-not-fried buffalo chicken wings still have all the spicy, saucy goodness of regular wings, but with fewer calories. Served with our homemade blue cheese dressing, this is your favorite bar food—only better!

SERVES 4 (FOR APPETIZERS)
Calories per serving, wings: 263
Calories per serving, blue cheese dressing: 226

For the wings:
- 1¼ pounds chicken wings, wing tips discarded, wings separated between first and second joints
- ½ cup low-sodium, low-fat chicken stock
- 2 tablespoons hot sauce (preferably Frank's), or more to taste
- 1 clove garlic, minced
  Pinch salt
- 1 tablespoon cornstarch

For the blue-cheese dressing:
- ⅓ cup nonfat buttermilk
- ⅓ cup reduced-fat mayonnaise
- ½ cup crumbled blue cheese
- 2 teaspoons lemon juice
  Pinch each salt and pepper

1. FOR THE WINGS, preheat the oven to 425 degrees, and arrange a rack in the center of the oven.

2. BRING 1 inch of water to a simmer in a large pot. Place the wings in a steamer basket, set it on top of the simmering water, cover, and steam 10 minutes. Drain on paper towels.

3. LINE a baking sheet with parchment paper. Arrange the wings in a single layer on the lined baking sheet and roast 20 minutes. Turn and continue roasting until well browned, and crisp, 15 to 20 more minutes.

4. MEANWHILE, combine the stock, hot sauce, garlic, and salt in a small saucepan. In a small bowl, stir the cornstarch with 1 tablespoon of water. Bring the hot-sauce mixture to a simmer, and stir in enough of the cornstarch mixture to thicken the sauce to the consistency of heavy cream (you'll use almost all of the cornstarch). Remove from the heat. Taste and add more hot sauce, if you like.

5. FOR THE DRESSING, combine all of the ingredients in a blender and blend until smooth.

6. WHEN THE WINGS ARE COOKED, transfer to a bowl. Return the hot-sauce mixture to a simmer, pour over the wings, and toss to coat. Serve with the dressing.

Tips

1. Traditional, high-calorie buffalo wings are deep-fried to make them crunchy. These are roasted, with no added oil, but first they are steamed. This technique not only gets rid of some of the fat, but it makes them brown and crisp better during roasting. Line the baking sheet with parchment paper, not aluminum foil—the wings will stick to foil.

2. The traditional sauce is made with melted butter flavored with hot sauce. This recipe replaces the butter with chicken stock, thickened with a little cornstarch.

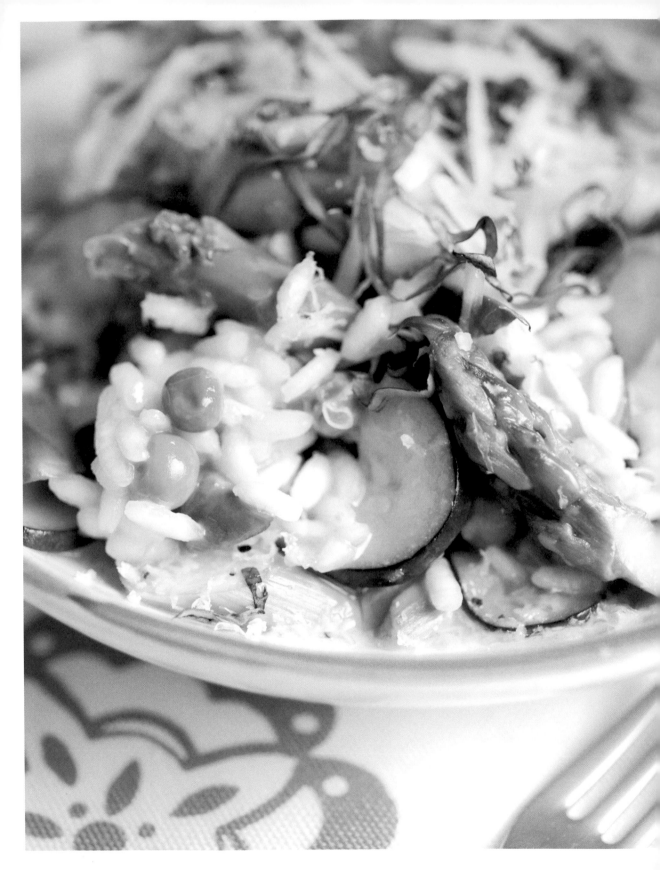

Risotto with Spring Vegetables

It takes a little stirring, but the effort pays off every time when you sit down to a plate of creamy rice and vegetables. The luxurious texture comes from the rice grains themselves with little added fat, and there's plenty of room for as many veggies as you desire.

SERVES 4
Calories per serving: 489

1	tablespoon olive oil
¼	cup chopped onion
1	clove garlic, chopped
2	medium (about 12 ounces) zucchini, trimmed, halved lengthwise, sliced ¼- to ⅓-inch thick
4½ to 5 cups low-sodium chicken broth	
1	pound medium asparagus, ends trimmed
½	cup frozen peas, thawed
¼	cup grated Parmesan cheese
2	tablespoons thinly sliced basil
¾	teaspoon salt
1	tablespoon unsalted butter
1½	cups short-grain rice (Arborio or Carnaroli)
½	cup dry white wine
¼	teaspoon pepper
2	tablespoons chopped mint (optional), for garnish

1. COMBINE the oil and onion in a large saucepan over medium heat and cook, stirring occasionally, until the onion is translucent, 2 to 3 minutes. Add the garlic and cook 1 minute. Add the zucchini, turn the heat to medium-low, and cook until softened and lightly browned, 18 to 20 minutes.

2. MEANWHILE, bring the 5 cups stock to a simmer in a saucepan wide enough to hold the asparagus. Add the asparagus and simmer until barely tender, about 3 minutes. Remove with a slotted spoon or tongs. Cut off the tips in nice sized pieces (about 1½ inches), and cut the stalks into smaller, bite-sized pieces; transfer to a bowl. Add the peas, ¼ cup of the cheese, and 1 tablespoon basil; set aside. Put a lid over the stock, and reduce the heat to very low so that the stock barely simmers.

3. WHEN THE ZUCCHINI IS COOKED, stir in ½ teaspoon salt, and the remaining 1 tablespoon of the basil. Add the butter and the rice, increase

the heat to medium-high, and cook, stirring with a wooden spoon, until the rice is translucent, 1 to 2 minutes. Add the wine and cook, stirring, until most of the liquid has evaporated, about 1 minute. Add $\frac{1}{2}$ cup simmering stock and cook, stirring frequently, until most of the liquid has been absorbed, about 2 minutes. Continue adding the broth, about $\frac{1}{2}$ cup at a time, and cooking, stirring frequently, until the rice is just tender and the mixture is creamy and has the texture of loose porridge, 17 to 20 minutes. The rice mixture should bubble away at a good clip. (You may not use all of the stock.) Stir in the reserved contents of the bowl and season with the remaining $\frac{1}{4}$ teaspoon salt, and the pepper.

Tips

1. Risotto relies on the combination of the starch released from special varieties of short-grain Italian rice, such as Arborio, mixed with liquid (usually broth), and fat, to create a creamy, clinging sauce which bathes the rice.

2. With less than half the usual oil, butter, and cheese, this recipe is quite a bit less rich than the traditional, but slow-cooked zucchini contributes to a soft, silky texture. Additional vegetables add bulk in place of fat, and other vegetables (such as fennel, butternut squash, spinach, and mushrooms) can be added, or substituted for those used below.

3. We like using lots of different veggies, but if it's too complicated, cut the asparagus, and double the zucchini.

Stuffed Portobello Mushrooms

The mouthfeel of steak without the fat, portobellos curb carnivorous meat cravings without compromising flavor. And stuffed with garlic, herbs, and a little fontina cheese, these caps will become a regular visitor to your cocktail hour or dinner table.

SERVES 4
Calories per serving: 329

4	portobello mushrooms, stems removed
3	garlic cloves, minced
1	tablespoon balsamic vinegar
2	tablespoons olive oil
1	cup fresh whole wheat breadcrumbs
¼	cup finely chopped fresh flat-leaf parsley
¼	cup finely chopped fresh basil
	Salt and pepper
¼	cup crumbled fontina cheese

1. PREHEAT the broiler. Using a spoon, scrape out the mushroom gills. Place mushrooms in a shallow dish. Whisk together garlic, vinegar, and 1 tablespoon oil, and pour over mushrooms, turning to coat. Transfer to a rimmed baking sheet and broil, turning once and brushing with remaining marinade occasionally, until softened and cooked through, about 10 minutes.

2. WHILE THE MUSHROOMS ARE COOKING, in a bowl, combine bread-crumbs, parsley, basil, remaining tablespoon oil, ½ teaspoon salt, and ¼ teaspoon pepper.

3. REMOVE the mushrooms from the oven, sprinkle with ¼ teaspoon salt and ¼ teaspoon pepper. Sprinkle 1 tablespoon cheese into the cavity of each of the mushroom caps. Return to the broiler and broil until cheese melts, about 1 minute. Spread ¼ cup breadcrumb mixture over the cheese in each of the mushroom caps, and broil until toasted and golden brown, about 2 minutes. Serve immediately.

Marinated Lamb Kebabs with Yogurt Sauce

Lamb gets the royal Mediterranean treatment in these juicy kebabs redolent with smoky spices and spiked with lemon, pine nuts, and dried apricot. Crunchy slaw and a garlicky yogurt sauce are the finishing touches to this riot of low-fat flavor.

SERVES 4
Calories per serving: 369
Calories per serving, pita: 85

For the lamb:
1	large garlic clove
1/4	teaspoon salt
1	teaspoon ground cumin
1	teaspoon ground coriander
1	teaspoon ground turmeric
1/2	teaspoon paprika
1/4	cup mixed pine nuts, pistachios and chopped dried apricots
2	teaspoons lemon juice
1	tablespoon olive oil
1/2	teaspoon honey
2	tablespoons tomato paste
3/4	pound one-inch cubed leg of lamb (trimmed of all visible fat)

For the salad:
1	cup iceberg lettuce, shredded
1	cup purple cabbage
4	tomatoes, sliced thinly

For the dressing:
4	heaping tablespoons low-fat Greek yogurt
2	heaping tablespoons mayonnaise
1	clove garlic, minced

Optional:
2 whole wheat pitas, sliced in half

1. COMPLETELY COVER and soak eight bamboo skewers in cold water.

2. GRIND the garlic and salt in a food processor. Once the mixture has turned to paste, add the ground cumin, coriander, turmeric, paprika, pine nuts, pistachios, and dried apricots, and grind again to mix thoroughly.

3. ADD the mixture into a medium-sized bowl and combine with the lemon juice, olive oil, honey, and tomato paste.

4. ADD the cubed lamb to the paste and coat the meat completely. Cover with plastic wrap and marinate 20 minutes to two hours. While the meat is marinating, make the salad and the dressing.

5. FOR THE SALAD, toss together the shredded cabbage and lettuce.

6. FOR THE DRESSING, mix together the yogurt, mayonnaise, and minced garlic.

7. DRAIN the bamboo skewers and pat dry. Thread four pieces of lamb onto each bamboo stick.

8. HEAT grill pan so that it is hot, but not smoking. Cook the meat for 4 minutes on each of its 4 sides, turning them carefully. Once the meat is all cooked, remove and allow it to rest for 5 minutes under aluminum foil.

9. WHILE THE MEAT IS RESTING, place the pita bread in the toaster for a minute to puff the pita without toasting it. Once puffed up, cut along one side with a pair of scissors and open the hot pita pocket up. Repeat this step with the remaining pitas.

10. SPREAD a couple of tablespoons of the yogurt dressing into each of the pitas. Add the cooked meat from one or two skewers by easing it off the sticks with a fork. Add a handful of salad and a few tomato slices.

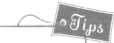

Tips

1. The longer you leave the lamb to marinate, the more flavorful it will be.

....

2. It is important that your grill pan is not so hot that you burn the honey and the garlic in the marinade but hot enough to create grill marks.

....

3. You can leave out the pita and eat the lamb kebabs straight from the sticks. In this case, toss the salad in the dressing to coat and serve alongside the kebabs.

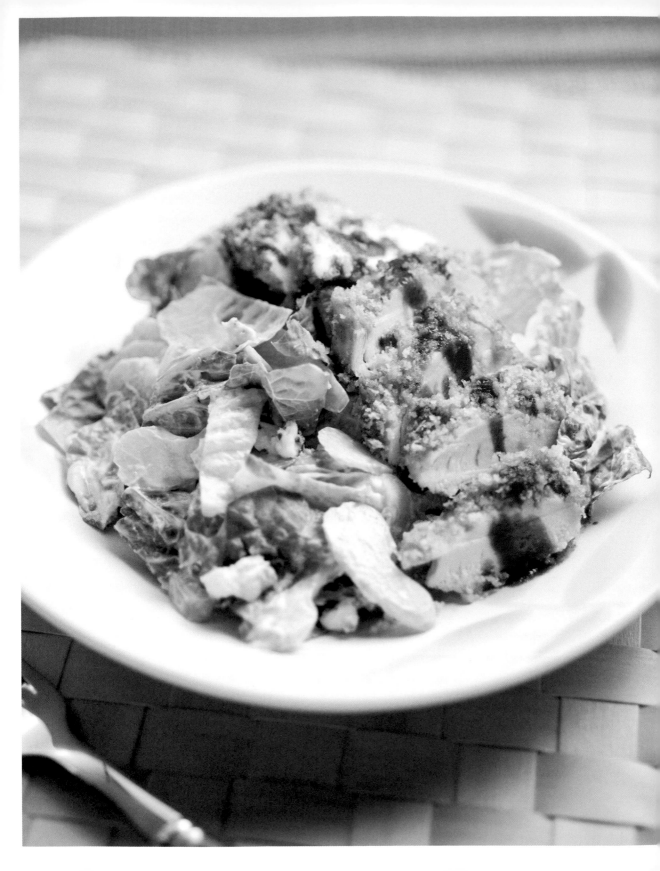

Buffalo Chicken Salad

Chicken tenders baked in a crunchy crust peel away most of the fat and mess of actually deep frying buffalo wings. The super fattening melted butter sauce of the original is gone too, and we've swapped the full-fat dressing for low- or no-fat buttermilk and yogurt sprinkled with tasty blue cheese.

SERVES 4
Calories per serving: 480

2	tablespoons hot sauce (preferably Frank's)
1	teaspoon apple cider vinegar
1	teaspoon dark brown sugar
¼	teaspoon salt
1	pound chicken tenders
½	cup whole wheat breadcrumbs or Panko
1	teaspoon vegetable oil
1	ounce crumbled blue cheese (about ¼ cup)
¼	cup plain nonfat yogurt
2	tablespoons nonfat or low-fat buttermilk
¼	teaspoon black pepper.
1	head romaine lettuce, chopped
6	celery stalks, thinly sliced

1. PREHEAT the oven to 400 degrees. Whisk together the hot sauce, vinegar, sugar, and salt in a shallow dish until well blended. Add the chicken and turn to coat. Marinate for 10 minutes at room temperature.

2. PUT the breadcrumbs and oil in a shallow dish and toss to combine. Dredge each chicken tender in the breadcrumbs, completely coating both sides. Transfer to the rack of a broiler pan or to a metal rack fitted over a rimmed baking sheet. Bake, turning once, until chicken is cooked through and crust is golden brown, about 12 minutes.

3. WHILE THE CHICKEN IS BAKING, stir together the cheese, yogurt, buttermilk, and pepper. Toss with the lettuce and celery until well coated. Divide the dressed greens and chicken tenders among 4 serving plates and serve immediately.

Tuna Salad Rolls with Edamame

In some parts of the country, Boston lettuce is known as "butter lettuce" and it's pretty obvious why in these light and naturally sweet tuna salad rolls. We love everything about them: putting them together, dipping them in the tangy ginger soy, and tasting all the clean flavors—in one crunchy bite.

SERVES 2
Calories per serving, tuna rolls: 269
Calories per serving, cucumber salad: 38
Calories per serving, dipping sauce: 30
Calories per serving, edamame: 97

For the marinated cucumber salad:
1   cucumber, peeled, and sliced thin
$\frac{1}{4}$ cup rice wine vinegar
$\frac{1}{4}$ teaspoon salt
1   teaspoon sugar
1   teaspoon sesame seeds, toasted in a dry skillet over low heat until fragrant, 3 to 5 minutes

For the dipping sauce:
$\frac{1}{4}$ cup rice wine vinegar
2   tablespoons low-sodium soy sauce
1   teaspoon toasted sesame oil
1   rounded teaspoon slivered fresh ginger

For the edamame:
3   cups frozen edamame in the shell
$1\frac{1}{2}$ teaspoons salt, for water
$\frac{1}{2}$ teaspoon kosher salt, to taste

For assembly:
7   ounces water-packed albacore tuna, drained
1   tablespoon olive oil
    Salt, to taste
    Pepper, to taste
4   leaves Boston lettuce, bottom ($\frac{1}{2}$ inch) core removed
2   small bunches cilantro
2   small bunches mint
2   red bell peppers, stemmed, seeded, cored, and cut into thin strips
2   cups broccoli sprouts
8   scallions, trimmed and cut into 3-inch sections, thick ends split in half lengthwise

1. FOR THE CUCUMBERS, toss the cucumber with the vinegar and salt in a bowl; set aside while you prepare the rest of the recipe. Just before serving, stir in the sugar and sesame seeds.

2. FOR THE DIPPING SAUCE, stir together the ingredients in a small bowl; set aside.

3. FOR THE TUNA, in a small bowl, combine the tuna and olive oil, and season lightly with salt and pepper.

4. ARRANGE lettuce, herbs, bell pepper, sprouts, and scallions on a platter.

5. TO MAKE EACH ROLL, overlap 2 lettuce leaves on a plate, stem ends facing up. Arrange 4 sprigs cilantro, and 3 to 4 mint leaves horizontally in the center of the overlapped lettuce leaves. Spoon about one-eighth of the tuna on top. Arrange 3 to 4 pepper strips, and some of the scallions, horizontally on top, leaving 1 to 1 1/2 inches of the lettuce free at the bottom. Add about 1 tablespoon sprouts. Spoon some of the dipping sauce over. Fold the bottom of the lettuce up over the tuna and vegetables. Fold in the right side, and roll to the left to make a roll, open at the top. Spoon a little more of the dipping sauce onto the open top, and eat immediately over a plate to catch juices.

6. TO MAKE THE EDAMAME: Bring 4 cups of water to a boil in a saucepan, add edamame and 1 teaspoon salt, and boil for 4 minutes. Drain and sprinkle with 1/2 teaspoon of kosher salt.

Tips

1. Lettuce leaves and a virtually fat-free dipping sauce replace bread and mayonnaise.

2. Look for edamame in the frozen vegetable section of your supermarket.

Huevos Rancheros

All the fantastic tastes of Mexico meet for breakfast in this classic dish that's naturally easy on the waistline. Big flavors rule the day as spiced up tomato, guacamole, and black beans with chipotle all get together alongside eggs, yogurt, and cheese to create a fiesta on a plate.

SERVES 4
Calories per serving: 503

For the ranchero sauce:
- 1 (14- to 15-ounce) can whole peeled tomatoes in juice
- 1/2 cup coarsely chopped red or white onion
- 1/2 jalapeño pepper, stemmed, seeded (or not, if you like heat), coarsely chopped
- 1 garlic clove, coarsely chopped
- 2 teaspoons olive oil
- 1 green or red bell pepper (or 1/2 each), cut into strips
- 1/2 teaspoon ground cumin
- 1 tablespoon chopped cilantro, plus extra leaves, for garnish
  Salt

For the black beans:
- 1 (14- to 15- ounce) can black beans, drained
- 3/4 to 1 cup canned chicken stock
- 1/2 canned chipotle chile in adobo, seeded, and chopped, with about 1/2 teaspoon adobo
- 2 tablespoons chopped cilantro

For the guacamole:
- 1 ripe avocado, halved, seeded, and skinned
  Juice of 1/2 lime (about 4 teaspoons)
- 1/2 cup coarsely chopped cherry tomatoes
- 1/4 cup chunky (1/4 to 1/2 inch) chopped red onion
- 8 sprigs fresh cilantro, leaves and slender stems chopped
  Pinch salt

- 8 (5-inch) corn tortillas
- 2 teaspoons olive oil
- 4 large eggs
  Salt and pepper
- 2 scallions, chopped
- 2 ounces queso fresco, feta, or fresh goat cheese, crumbled
- 1 lime, quartered
- 2/3 cup nonfat yogurt, seasoned with pinch each salt and pepper

1. FOR THE SAUCE, combine tomatoes with their juice, onion, jalapeño, and garlic in the bowl of a food processor and blend until smooth. Heat the oil in a saucepan over medium-low heat. Add the peppers, sprinkle with the cumin and 1/2 teaspoon salt, and cook, covered, until softened, about 5 minutes. Add the tomato mixture and simmer gently, partially covered until slightly thickened, 8 to 10 minutes.

2. MEANWHILE, combine the beans, ¾ cup stock, and chopped chipotle with adobo in another saucepan. Bring to a simmer. With a whisk or potato masher, mash about one-half of the beans until the mixture thickens. Remove from heat and stir in cilantro.

3. IN ANOTHER BOWL, use a fork to mash the avocado with the lime juice until the mixture is soft, but still very chunky. Add the tomatoes, onion, cilantro, and salt and stir to combine; set aside.

4. PREHEAT the oven to 250 degrees. Wrap tortillas loosely in aluminum foil and warm in the oven.

5. HEAT the oil in a 10-inch nonstick skillet over medium heat. Crack the eggs into the skillet, and reduce the heat to low. Sprinkle lightly with salt and pepper. Cover and cook 3 minutes until whites are set.

6. TO SERVE, re-warm salsa and beans, adding remaining stock to beans if they have thickened. Spoon salsa onto each of 4 plates. Overlap 2 tortillas on top of the salsa. Place a fried egg on top, and spoon more salsa on top. Divide the beans between the plates; sprinkle with cheese. Garnish with guacamole, yogurt, chopped scallion, and cilantro leaves. Serve with lime.

> **Tip**
>
> Canned black beans, heated and mashed with chicken stock, make a low-fat alternative to refried beans. Seasoned nonfat yogurt stands in for sour cream. Use store-bought guacamole, if you like.

Asian Beef Noodle Soup

This take-off on Pho, a traditional Vietnamese noodle soup, gives you all of the comfort of a hot lunch without all the calories! Brimming with thinly sliced steak, noodles, vegetables, and herbs, this is truly a one-bowl wonder.

SERVES 4
Calories per serving: 482

For the broth:

4   cups chicken or beef broth
4   cups water
2   thin slices peeled ginger
2   whole pieces star anise
1   small ($\frac{1}{2}$-inch) section cinnamon stick
$\frac{1}{4}$ shallot, thinly sliced
2   tablespoons low-sodium soy sauce, plus extra for serving
$\frac{1}{8}$ teaspoon pepper

For the garnish:

8   ounces dried Asian rice noodles
$\frac{1}{2}$ pound boneless beef sirloin, or London broil, trimmed of any fat, frozen
1   small head romaine lettuce, shredded, or 2 cups shredded Savoy cabbage
1   rounded cup bean sprouts
1   red or green bell pepper, seeded, stemmed, and thinly sliced
3   scallions, minced
$\frac{1}{2}$ cup thinly sliced radish
1   cup fresh cilantro sprigs (pluck off the top leaves with slender stem attached)
$\frac{1}{2}$ jalapeño pepper, seeded, stemmed, and minced
$\frac{1}{2}$ cup fresh basil leaves
$\frac{1}{4}$ cup fresh mint leaves
    Salt
2   tablespoons peanuts, chopped
    Lime wedges, for garnish
    Toasted sesame oil, for serving
    Hoisin sauce, for serving

1. FOR THE COOKING LIQUID, in a large saucepan, bring the broth, water, ginger, star anise, cinnamon, and shallot to a boil. Reduce heat to very low, partially cover, and simmer 15 minutes; remove spices with a slotted spoon. Add soy sauce and pepper, set aside.

2. MEANWHILE, in a large bowl, soak noodles in cold water to cover until softened and pliable, 30 minutes. Bring a large pot of salted water to a boil.

3. WITH A VERY SHARP KNIFE, cut uncooked beef across the grain into very thin slices; arrange on a serving plate and refrigerate until ready to serve. Arrange all of the other vegetables, herbs, chopped peanuts, and lime wedges on a second, large platter.

4. DRAIN noodles in a colander. Add to boiling water and cook, stirring, 45 seconds. Drain noodles again.

5. TO SERVE, bring broth to a boil. Divide steak slices between 4 large serving bowls. Ladle broth over noodles. Add noodles, vegetables and herbs to each bowl. Everyone can season their soup with lime wedges, salt, soy sauce, sesame oil, and/or hoisin sauce, as they like.

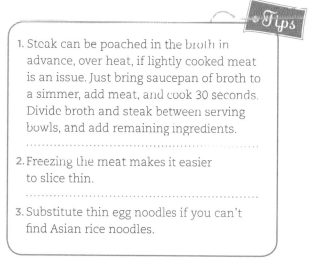

Tips

1. Steak can be poached in the broth in advance, over heat, if lightly cooked meat is an issue. Just bring saucepan of broth to a simmer, add meat, and cook 30 seconds. Divide broth and steak between serving bowls, and add remaining ingredients.

2. Freezing the meat makes it easier to slice thin.

3. Substitute thin egg noodles if you can't find Asian rice noodles.

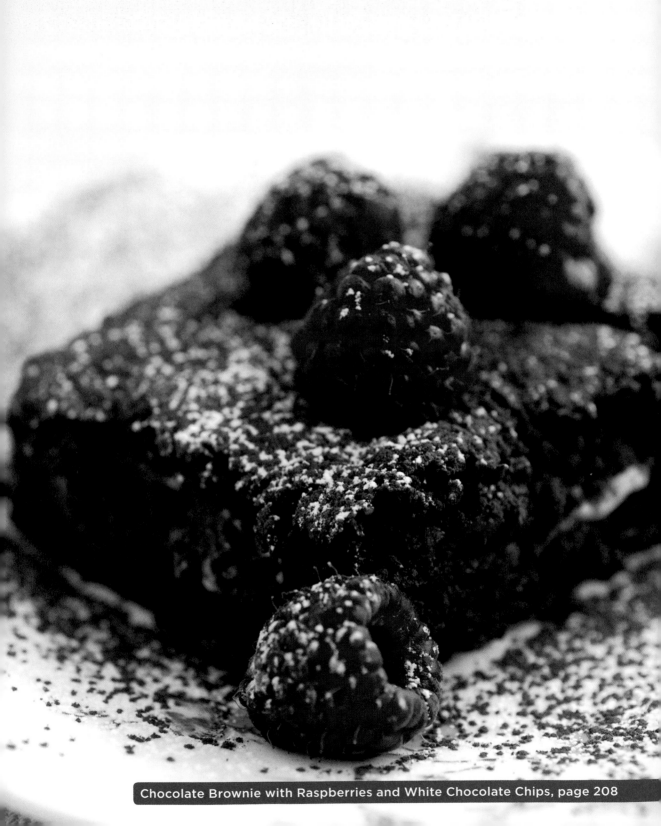

Chocolate Brownie with Raspberries and White Chocolate Chips, page 208

Sweets

Deep Dark Chocolate Cake

A little black coffee, ground almond, and tangy buttermilk add an air of mystery to this deeply chocolate cake. Grated beet (surprise!) is this cake's special secret, and is a healthy way to push the sweetness and cut the calories.

SERVES 10
Calories per serving: 222

For the cake:
- cooking spray
- 1½ cups self-rising flour
- ¼ cup finely ground almonds
- 5 tablespoons cocoa powder
- 1 teaspoon baking soda
- ¼ teaspoon salt
- 4 ounces beets, peeled and finely grated
- 4 ounces low-fat buttermilk
- 2 tablespoons strong black coffee
- 3 large eggs
- ¾ cup sugar

For the icing:
- ½ cup dark chocolate, cut into small pieces
- 2 tablespoons strong black coffee
- 2 tablespoons honey

For the top (optional):
Organic, unsprayed rose petals

1. **PREHEAT** the oven to 350 degrees.

2. **LIGHTLY SPRAY** an 8" springform baking pan with cooking spray

3. **IN A SMALL BOWL,** combine the flour, cocoa powder, ground almonds, salt, and baking soda onto a plate and set aside.

4. **USING A STANDING OR HANDHELD MIXER** using a medium speed, beat the eggs and sugar for 4 full minutes until pale and fluffy. On low speed, beat the beets, followed by dry ingredients. Add the buttermilk and coffee until the batter is smooth.

5. **POUR** into the pan and place in the middle of a hot oven and bake for 30 minutes. Test with a toothpick inserted for doneness, it should come clean. Bake for an additional 5 minutes if needed.

6. **COOL** for 10 minutes or so in the pan and unmold onto cooling rack. Cool on a wire rack until cold.

7. **TO MAKE THE ICING,** prepare a double boiler.

8. **COMBINE** all the ingredients and gently stir until the chocolate is smooth. Stir occasionally until the mixture thickens.

9. **WITH THE CAKE** still on the wire rack, pour the icing liberally over the top of the cake and let it drip down the sides. Transfer onto a plate or cake stand for serving and garnish with rose petals.

Tip

If you can't purchase finely ground almonds, pulse blanched almonds in a food processor until they resemble cornmeal. Do not over process or they will turn into nut butter.

Oatmeal Parfait

Versatile oatmeal takes a decidedly dessert turn in this fruity, sweet and cinnamony parfait that feels a lot like cheating—but isn't. Light yogurt reins in the fat without compromising your need for something creamy and satisfying.

SERVES 4
Calories per serving: 473

1   pound peaches, pitted, and cut into eighths
1   pound (6) plums, pitted and quartered
6   ounces blueberries
½   teaspoon ground cinnamon
    Salt
2   tablespoons maple syrup, plus 4 teaspoons, for drizzling
1   tablespoon orange juice
1¼ cups quick-cooking McCann's steel cut oatmeal
¼   cup nonfat or low-fat yogurt
2   tablespoons chopped pecans

1. **PREHEAT** the oven to 450 degrees. Arrange rack in top third of the oven.

2. **PLACE THE PEACHES,** plums, and blueberries in a 9-by-13-inch baking dish. Sprinkle with the cinnamon and a pinch of salt. Add the maple syrup and orange juice; toss with a rubber spatula to coat. Roast until the fruit is tender, 25 to 30 minutes.

3. **MEANWHILE,** cook the oatmeal according to package directions.

4. **TO ASSEMBLE,** using about half of the total quantity of oatmeal, spoon a layer of oatmeal into the bottoms of four serving bowls. Using about half of the fruit, spoon warm fruit and juices over the oatmeal. Top with the rest of the oatmeal, and then the rest of the fruit. Spoon a dollop of yogurt on top of each, drizzle with a little more maple syrup, and sprinkle with pecans.

Peanut Butter Dream Bars

Put down that jar! Go ahead and pinch yourself if you'd like, but you're not dreaming. These tasty peanut butter bars will satisfy several cravings at once and do it without breaking the fat bank.

SERVES 8
Calories per serving: 157

1/2   cup low-calorie thin chocolate wafers,
        finely ground in a food processor
1/2   cup old-fashioned oats
1/3   cup confectioners' sugar
1/2   teaspoon salt
3   tablespoons unsalted butter, melted and cooled
1/4   cup creamy reduced-fat peanut butter
1 1/2 ounces reduced-fat cream cheese, room temperature
2   teaspoons pure vanilla extract
2   tablespoons semi-sweet chocolate chips, melted

1. LINE a 9-by-4-inch loaf pan with wax paper or baking parchment leaving a 2-inch overhang on the long sides.

2. COMBINE the ground wafers, oats, sugar, and 1/4 teaspoon salt in a medium bowl. Stir in the butter until everything is evenly moistened. Stir in 1 tablespoon peanut butter until mixture forms large clumps. Transfer mixture to lined loaf pan and press into an even layer. Refrigerate until firm, about 10 minutes.

3. MEANWHILE, beat cream cheese with an electric mixer on medium speed until smooth and fluffy, about 2 minutes. Add vanilla, remaining 3 tablespoons peanut butter, and remaining 1/4 teaspoon salt, and beat on medium speed until pale and nearly doubled in volume, about 7 minutes. Transfer to the loaf pan and spread in an even layer over cookie crust. Freeze until firm, about 10 minutes.

4. SPREAD the chocolate in a thin, even layer over the chilled peanut butter layer. Refrigerate until firm, about 10 minutes. When ready to serve, lift bars out of the pan using the wax paper overhang. Cut crosswise into 8 bars and serve cold.

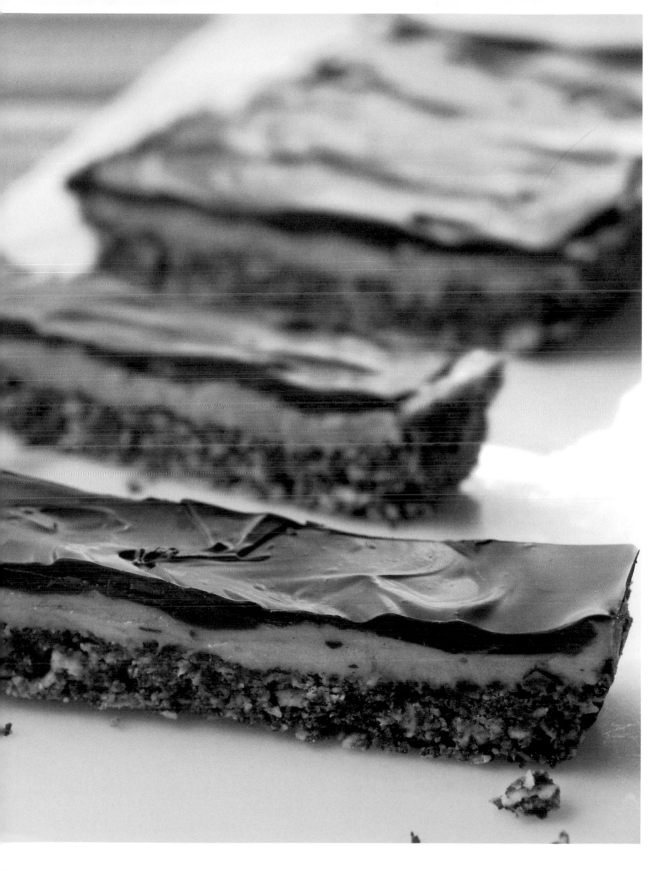

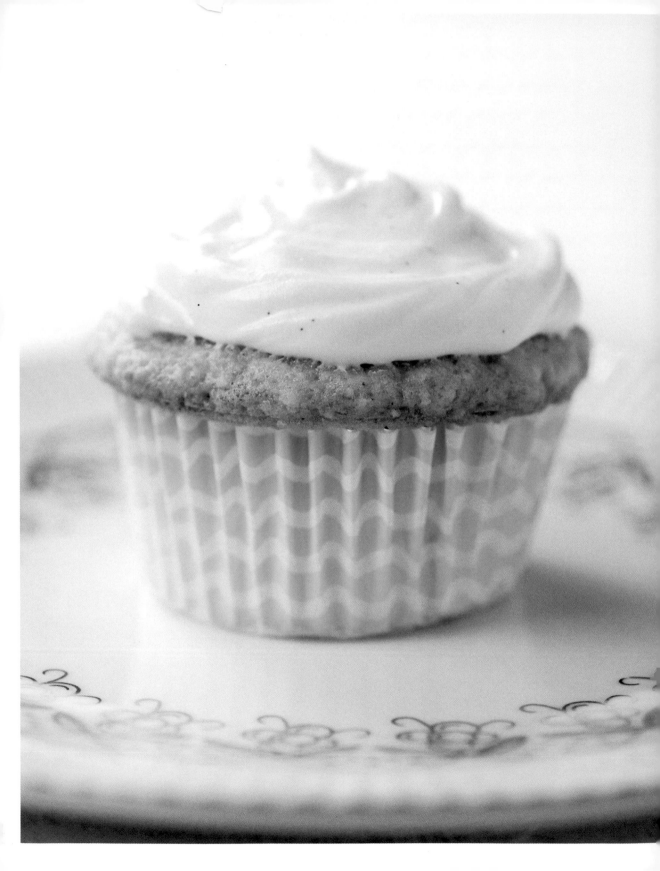

Vanilla Cupcakes

Zucchini wins the award for most unlikely appearance in a delicious treat, and gets glowing reviews for the texture and no-fat heft it brings to these sweet beauties. Go ahead, grab a cupcake—you deserve it!

MAKES 12 CUPCAKES
Calories per serving: 204

For the frosting:

3   large egg whites
1   cup sugar
    Pinch salt
¾   teaspoon vanilla extract
    Finely grated zest of ½ lemon

For the cupcakes:

1¼ cups all-purpose flour
½   cup finely ground almonds
1½ teaspoons baking powder
¼   teaspoon salt
2   large eggs
¾   cup sugar
2   teaspoons vanilla extract
1¼ cups peeled zucchini, finely grated

1. **PREHEAT** the oven to 350 degrees.

2. **TO MAKE THE FROSTING:** Combine the egg whites, sugar, salt, and vanilla extract in a heatproof bowl set over (not in) a pan of simmering water. Stir continuously over heat until the mixture is warm and the sugar is completely dissolved, 1 to 2 minutes.

3. **REMOVE** the bowl from the heat. Using a handheld electric or standing mixer set on high, beat until the mixture is entirely cooled, glossy, and stiff, about 7 minutes. Blend in the lemon zest until smooth—once smooth, take care not to over beat or the mixture will get lumpy. Let frosting set and cool in the refrigerator (at least 30 minutes), while making the cupcakes.

4. **TO MAKE THE CUPCAKES:** Arrange a rack in the center of the oven. Line a 12-muffin pan with cupcake liners.

5. **IN A BOWL,** whisk together the flour, almonds, and baking powder; set aside. In another bowl, beat the eggs, sugar, salt, and vanilla with a handheld or standing mixer until thick and light colored, about 4 minutes. Beat in the zucchini on low speed until fully incorporated.

6. ADD the dry ingredients and beat on low speed until fully incorporated, scraping down the bowl once with a spatula during beating. Use a $\frac{1}{3}$-cup measure to spoon into the muffin cups.

7. BAKE until a toothpick inserted into the center comes out clean, about 20 to 25 minutes, turning the pan midway through baking. Transfer cupcakes out onto a wire rack and cool completely before icing with the chilled frosting.

Chocolate Pudding

Try this simple chocolate pudding once and it will never leave your dessert repertoire. 1% milk keeps things on the right path and lets you enjoy this moment of quintessential decadence without guilt.

SERVES 4
Calories per serving: 199

1/4 cup sugar
1/4 cup Dutch process cocoa powder
3 tablespoons cornstarch
1/4 teaspoon salt
2 cups 1% milk
1 1/2 ounces bittersweet chocolate
1 teaspoon pure vanilla extract

1. **WHISK** together sugar, cocoa, cornstarch, and salt in a medium saucepan. Set over medium heat and add the milk in a slow, steady stream, whisking constantly.

2. **CONTINUE WHISKING** while bringing the mixture to a bare simmer, about 5 minutes. Add the chocolate and whisk until melted, about 3 minutes.

3. **REMOVE** from the heat, whisk in the vanilla extract, and divide among 4 serving dishes. Chill, uncovered, until set, about 3 hours. Serve cold.

Red Velvet Cupcakes

We think red velvet cake is the most alluring and mysterious of all sweets, and we really love the way it looks. Beets and red food coloring send the hue of these moist cupcakes into the stratosphere, and a touch of cocoa adds an intriguing hint of chocolate.

MAKES 12 CUPCAKES
Calories per serving: 212

For the cupcakes:

3	large eggs
$^3/_4$	cup sugar
$^1/_2$	cup beets, raw, peeled and finely grated
1	cup white flour
$^1/_2$	cup ground almonds
2	teaspoons baking powder
1	teaspoon red food coloring
2	teaspoons cocoa powder
$^1/_3$	cup buttermilk
$^1/_4$	teaspoon salt

For the icing:

1$^1/_2$	cups confectioners' sugar
4	teaspoons water
2	teaspoons vanilla extract
$^1/_4$	teaspoon cream of tartar
1	medium egg white
	Small pinch salt

1. **PREHEAT** the oven to 350 degrees. Line a 12-hole muffin tray with cupcake liners.

2. **IN A LARGE MIXING BOWL,** add the eggs, sugar, and salt, and using a handheld or standing mixer, beat on medium high for about 5 minutes, until pale and doubled in size.

3. **ADD** the grated beets, flour, ground almonds, cocoa powder, and baking powder. Stir to combine.

4. **ADD** the buttermilk and food coloring and beat again to make sure that all the ingredients are well incorporated.

5. **SPOON** into the cupcake liners, taking care not to fill more than two-thirds of the way up or it will overflow when cooking.

6. **BAKE** for 30 minutes.

7. **WHILE THE CUPCAKES ARE COOKING, MAKE THE ICING:** Prepare a double boiler.

8. PLACE all the ingredients in the bowl, and stir to dissolve the sugar with a clean metal spoon for exactly 4 minutes; the mixture should be warm.

9. REMOVE the bowl from the heat and beat with a hand or standing mixer on high speed, until cool and the mixture has turned into a meringue, no more than 5 minutes.

10. THE MIXTURE IS READY to use when it has formed stiff peaks.

11. PIPE OR SPREAD 1 heaping tablespoon of the icing over the cooled cupcakes, and take care to ice the cakes very quickly as the icing will start to set and is best when just made.

Tips

1. To keep cupcakes fresh a few days, store them in an air-tight container.

2. Don't allow the water in the double boiler to boil. It must be simmering or it will overcook the eggs in the icing.

Chocolate Brownie with Raspberries and White Chocolate Chips

These gorgeous brownies are both sophisticated and elegant with 2 types of chocolate and colorful raspberries. Butternut squash is the fat reducing secret ingredient.

SERVES 9
Calories per serving: 291

For the brownie:
1   heaping cup fresh raspberries
2   cups butternut squash, peeled and finely grated
½   cup white chocolate, chopped into small chunks
1   cup ground almonds
1¼ cups sugar
3   large eggs
¼   cup self-rising flour
½   cup Dutch process cocoa powder
1   teaspoon baking powder
¼   teaspoon salt

For the icing:
Cocoa powder, for garnish

1. PREHEAT the oven to 400 degrees.

2. LINE the pan with parchment paper. A big square placed over the top is enough, if you then cut into each corner to make a neat pleat. It's also a good idea to dot a tiny bit of oil on the base and sides to help the paper stick down.

3. ADD the eggs and sugar into a large bowl, and using a handheld or standing mixer, beat on medium high speed 4–5 minutes until pale, fluffy and quadrupled in size.

4. ADD the grated butternut squash and the flour, ground almonds, cocoa powder, salt and baking powder. Beat until well incorporated. Pour half of this mixture into the prepared tin. Scatter the raspberries and chocolate chips over the top. Top with remaining batter.

5. BAKE for 20 minutes until just cooked.

6. LET COOL in the pan for 20 minutes and garnish with sifted cocoa powder before serving.

Tips

1. Don't be alarmed that the brownie is quite undercooked when it comes out of the oven. The 20 minutes' cooling down time is just enough to set the cake to that perfect squidgy brownie-ness.

2. By all means, swap the white chocolate for milk or dark if you would prefer. This will by no means tamper with the method for this recipe.

Mint Chocolate Cupcakes

Mint and chocolate collide with delicious results in these easy low-fat cupcakes. We love the playfulness of shocking green icing contrasting with the sophisticated dark chocolate shavings in these cupcakes that feel at home on linen or in a lunch box.

MAKES 12 CUPCAKES
Calories per serving: 336

For the cupcakes:
2   large eggs
³⁄₄   cup sugar
1   heaped cup peeled and finely grated sweet potato
¹⁄₂   cup finely ground almonds
³⁄₄   cup plain flour
1   teaspoon peppermint extract
¹⁄₄   teaspoon salt
1   tablespoon Dutch process cocoa powder
2   teaspoons baking powder
³⁄₄   cup dark chocolate chips or mint chocolate bar cut into chunks

For the icing:
2   cups confectioners' sugar
2   ounces unsalted butter, room temperature
¹⁄₂   teaspoon green food coloring
1   teaspoon peppermint extract
2   tablespoons cold water

For the top:
Shavings of dark chocolate

1. **PREHEAT** the oven to 350 degrees. Line a 12-hole muffin pan with paper liners.

2. **USING A HANDHELD OR STANDING MIXER,** whisk the eggs and sugar for 5 minutes, until pale and quadrupled in size. Add the grated sweet potato and whisk again. Whisk in the ground almonds, flour, peppermint extract, salt, cocoa powder, and baking powder until they are well combined. Add the chocolate chunks or chips and using a spatula, mix so that they are evenly distributed.

3. **DIVIDE** the batter evenly between the cupcake liners so that each liner is half-filled. This will give them enough space to puff up and rise to the top while baking.

4. **BAKE** at 350 degrees for 20 minutes. They will be somewhat flat on top rather than dome shaped.

5. **ONCE COOKED,** remove from the oven and cool for 15 minutes. Transfer to the refrigerator until the cupcakes are cold. The cupcakes will need to be cold to keep the icing from sliding off.

6. **WHILE THE CUPCAKES ARE BAKING, MAKE THE ICING:** With a wooden spoon or mixer, beat the butter with one heaped tablespoon of the sugar, the peppermint extract and coloring for a minute until they are all incorporated and the butter has softened slightly. Add the confectioners' sugar one heaped tablespoon at a time, with half a teaspoon of water each time you add the sugar, and beat between each addition. Once all the sugar is added, you should have a soft green paste.

7. **ICE** each cold cupcake, using just over a tablespoon of frosting per cupcake. Finish by sprinkling dark chocolate shavings over the top of each one.

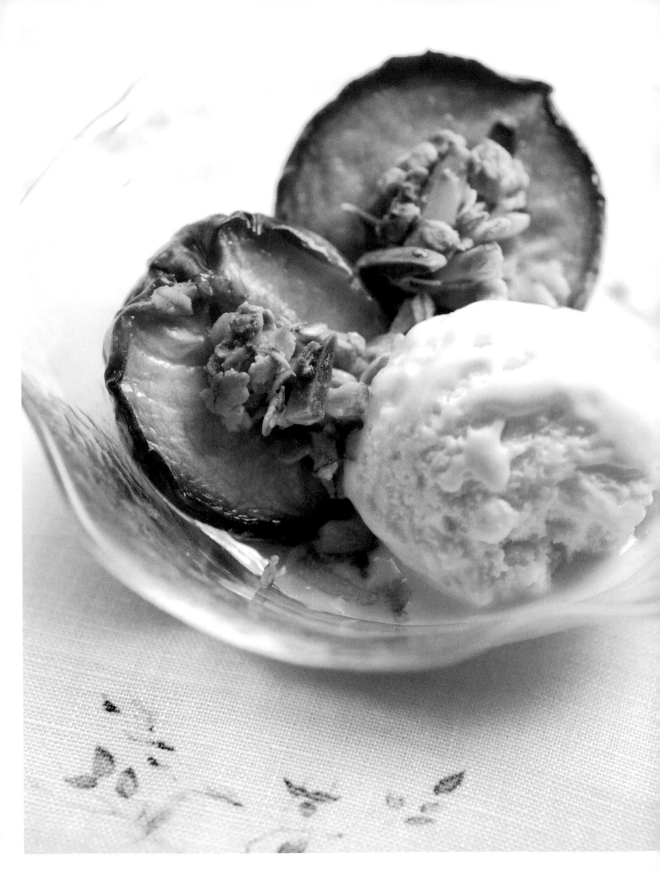

Roasted Peach Crisp

Ground cardamom is the real secret to this dessert. Its mysterious essence imbues the peaches with complex and haunting notes you really don't expect to find. Makes this crisp a real revelation.

SERVES 4
Calories per serving: 179

2	ripe peaches, halved and pitted
2	tablespoons honey
1	large egg white
2	tablespoons sugar
2	teaspoons vegetable oil
1/4	teaspoon salt
	Pinch of ground cardamom
1/3	cup slivered almonds
1/4	cup old-fashioned oats

1. **PREHEAT** oven to 425 degrees.

2. **ARRANGE** the peaches, cut side up, in a small glass or ceramic baking dish, and drizzle with honey. Pour 2 tablespoons water in the dish. Bake until tender and tops are caramelized, 30 to 40 minutes.

3. **MEANWHILE,** whisk together egg white, sugar, oil, salt, and cardamom until well blended. Stir in almonds and oats until evenly coated. Spread mixture in an even layer on a small, rimmed baking sheet. Place in the oven alongside the peaches and bake until golden brown, about 10 minutes. Remove from the oven and cool completely. (The mixture will crisp as it cools.)

4. **TRANSFER** each peach half to individual serving dishes. Break the almond mixture into large pieces, and arrange decoratively on peaches. Serve immediately.

Tip

Serve with low-fat vanilla ice cream or yogurt.

Chewy Oatmeal Raisin Cookies

These aren't the same old oatmeal cookies you grew up with. Not by a long shot. The whiskey and dark brown sugar guarantee that. Plus you lose a lot of the fat by replacing it with an all-fruit substitute, keeping the cookies moist without the usual compromises.

MAKES ABOUT 40 (2½-INCH) COOKIES
Calories per cookie: 116

2	tablespoons whiskey, or rum
⅔	cup raisins
8	tablespoons unsalted butter, at room temperature
¼	cup natural unsweetened applesauce
¾	cup firmly packed dark brown sugar
¾	cup granulated sugar
½	teaspoon salt
1	large egg
1	large egg white
¼	cup milk
2	teaspoons pure vanilla extract
2	cups all-purpose flour
1	teaspoon baking soda
½	teaspoon cinnamon
2	cups oats (not instant)

1. **SET** the oven rack in the middle position. Preheat the oven to 350 degrees. Line 2 baking sheets with parchment paper or spray with non-stick cooking spray; set aside.

2. **SPRINKLE** the whiskey or rum over the raisins in a bowl and let stand while you assemble the batter.

3. **USING A HANDHELD OR STANDING MIXER,** beat the butter, applesauce, brown sugar, granulated sugar, and salt on medium-high speed until light and fluffy, 2 to 3 minutes, scraping down the sides of the bowl halfway through. Beat in the egg and egg white, milk, and vanilla.

4. **IN A MEDIUM BOWL,** whisk together the flour, baking soda, and cinnamon, add to the batter, and beat just until the flour is absorbed. Gently fold in the oats with a rubber scraper.

5. USE 2 spoons to scoop out the batter by rounded teaspoonfuls onto the prepared baking sheets, 1½ inches apart. Bake until the cookies are set but still soft in the centers, and beginning to brown on the edges, 17 to 20 minutes.

6. LET cool on a wire rack.

Tip

Line the baking sheet with parchment paper instead of greasing with butter or oil; the paper adds no calories, keeps the cookies from sticking, and gets rid of the need to clean the baking sheet.

Iced Cappuccino Delight

Think a frothy iced cappuccino topped with sweet whipped cream is totally out of the question? Think again! All you have to do is bolster that healthy skim milk with a little fat-free yogurt and you've got something thick, delicious, and ready to dollop.

SERVES 4
Calories per serving: 110

For the cappuccino:
1   cup coffee, cooled or 2 shots espresso
1   cup skim milk
3   tablespoons fat-free plain Greek yogurt
5   tablespoons fat-free chocolate syrup
1   cup ice

For the whipped cream:
½   cup heavy cream
1   teaspoon confectioners' sugar

1. FOR THE CAPPUCCINO: Place the coffee, milk, yogurt, syrup, and ice in a blender and blend until desired.

2. FOR THE WHIPPED CREAM: In a large mixing bowl, beat the cream until soft peaks form. Add the confectioners' sugar. Continue to beat until stiff peaks form. At this point, you may add extracts or any additional flavorings you may like.

3. FOR THE ASSEMBLY: Pour the cappuccino in a glass and top with whipped cream. Garnish with a sprig of fresh mint.

Chocolate and Cranberry Biscotti

Delightful with coffee or just on their own, these crunchy cookies blend almond and cranberry with vanilla and a hint of chocolate for a sophisticated not-too-sweet treat. Best part—you can eat two without any guilt.

MAKES ABOUT 1 1/2 DOZEN
Calories per biscotti: 76

- 3/4 cup all-purpose flour
- 1/4 cup finely ground almonds
- 3 tablespoons Dutch-process cocoa powder
- 3/4 teaspoon baking powder
- 1/4 teaspoon salt
- 1 large egg
- 1/3 cup sugar
- 2 teaspoons pure vanilla extract
- 1/2 teaspoon almond extract
- 1/3 cup dried cranberries
  melted chocolate for drizzling

1. PREHEAT oven to 350 degrees and arrange a rack in the center of the oven. Line a baking sheet with parchment paper.

2. WHISK together flour, ground almonds, cocoa powder, baking powder, and salt in a medium bowl.

3. BEAT egg and sugar with a handheld or standing mixer on medium-high speed until pale and thick, about 5 minutes. Beat in vanilla and almond extracts. Reduce speed to low, and gradually add flour mixture. Beat until no traces of flour remain. Stir in cranberries. The dough will be very wet and sticky.

4. SCRAPE the dough in a thick line in the center of the prepared baking sheet. Wet your hands and pat dough into a 9-by-3-inch rectangle. Bake until puffed and dry to the touch, about 25 minutes. Cool on pan for 15 minutes; keep oven on. Peel off parchment and

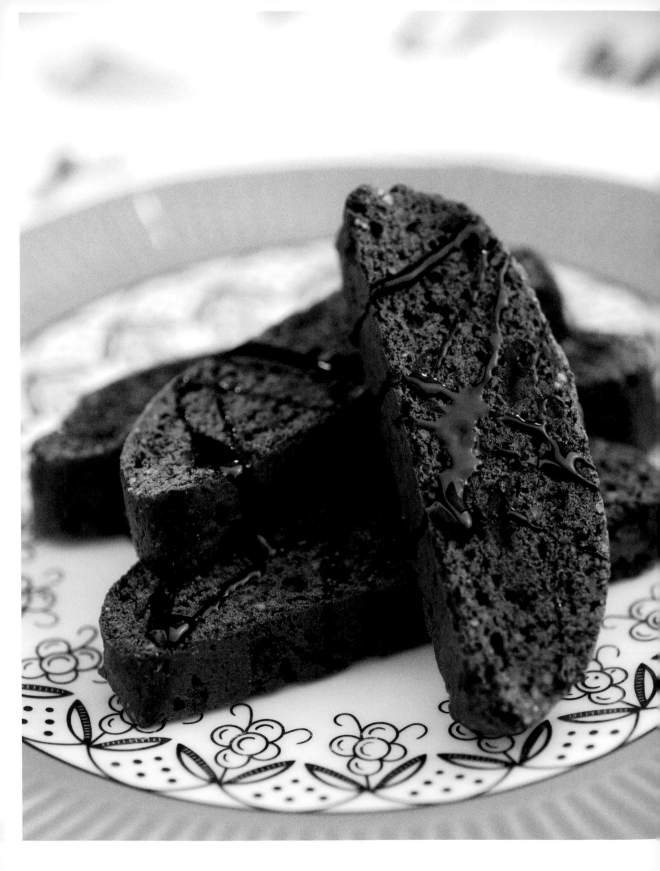

carefully transfer rectangle to a cutting board. Cut crosswise into $\frac{1}{3}$-inch-thick slices.

5. LAY slices flat on unlined baking sheet, and bake until dry, about 10 minutes. Flip slices and bake for 10 minutes more. Let cool completely. Cookies will crisp as they cool.

5. DRIZZLE with melted chocolate if desired.

1. Serve with low-fat vanilla ice cream or yogurt.

2. These cookies are very crisp, perfect for dunking in coffee or tea.

3. Cocoa powder gives the cookies the rich taste of chocolate with far fewer calories than chocolate chips or pieces, and virtually no fat.

Apple Cinnamon Cake

These traditional, comforting flavors come together in a wonderful way in this delicious and nutritious cake. Your friends won't believe you when you say the secret to this cake's fantastic texture is healthy white sweet potato. Healthy cake? They'll never suspect a thing.

SERVES 12
Calories per serving: 243

For the cake:
1   large apple (about 10 ounces)
     juice of 1 lemon
1¼ cups finely ground almonds
1   cup self-rising flour
1   teaspoon baking soda
¼   teaspoon salt
1   tablespoon ground cinnamon
3   large eggs
¾   cup superfine sugar
2   cups peeled sweet potato, finely grated (the white variety), grated at the very last minute to prevent discoloration
2   teaspoons vanilla extract

For the icing:
1   cup confectioners' sugar, sifted
4   tablespoons fresh lemon juice

1. PREHEAT the oven to 350 degrees. Grease the base and sides of an 8-inch springform pan with a little vegetable oil and a pastry brush. Line the pan with parchment paper.

2. PEEL, core and chop the apple into ¼ inch cubes. Toss them in a small bowl with some lemon juice to prevent oxidation.

3. IN A SEPARATE BOWL, combine the ground almonds, flour, baking soda, salt and cinnamon. Set aside.

4. IN A LARGE MIXING BOWL using a handheld or standing mixer, whisk together the eggs and sugar until pale and tripled in size, about 3 minutes on high speed. Add the grated sweet potato and whisk to combine. Lower the speed and add the dry ingredients to the bowl. Add the vanilla extract and mix. Using a rubber spatula, gently fold in the apple cubes.

5. POUR the batter into the prepared pan and bake for 30 minutes. Cover the top with aluminium foil and bake for an additional 30 minutes.

6. ONCE COOKED, cool on a wire rack for 10 minutes and make the icing.

7. TO MAKE THE ICING, stir the sifted sugar with the lemon juice. Drizzle liberally over the top of the cake, spreading with a knife to even out, and serve.

Carrot Cake

You always think carrot cake will be good for you until you taste the tons of fat in each bite. Well, here's a cake that actually lives up to the promise by being super low in fat. Sweet golden raisins, orange juice, and nuts team up to take this cake's spicy flavors over the top while classic cream cheese icing delivers a taste that screams "carrot cake."

SERVES 9
Calories per serving: 310

For the cake:
1	orange
1	lemon
$3/4$	cup golden raisins
3	medium eggs
$1 1/4$	cups light brown sugar
$2 1/2$	cups carrots, finely grated
1	cup self-rising flour
1	teaspoon cinnamon
$1/2$	teaspoon ground ginger
1	teaspoon baking soda
$1/4$	teaspoon salt
1	cup ground almonds
$1/4$	cup walnuts, roughly chopped

For the icing:
3	cups confectioners' sugar
$1/2$	cup full-fat cream cheese
1	teaspoon fresh lemon juice
	finely grated zest of $1/2$ lemon

1. **PREHEAT** the oven to 350 degrees.

2. **LINE** the base of an 8-inch square pan with parchment paper. Lightly brush over the base and sides with a little vegetable oil.

3. **GRATE** the zest of the orange and the lemon and set aside. Squeeze the orange juice into a bowl and add the golden raisins to the juice. Set aside.

4. **WHISK** the eggs and sugar with the orange and lemon zest using a handheld or standing mixer for five minutes until pale and full of air. Add the grated carrot and beat to incorporate.

5. **SLOWLY ADD** in the spices, salt, ground almonds, baking soda and flour, then quickly mix until all the ingredients are combined.

6. USING A SPATULA, mix in the golden raisins, along with any orange juice left in the bowl, along with the walnuts until they are evenly distributed.

7. POUR into the prepared pan and bake for 40 minutes.

8. WHEN A TOOTHPICK INSERTED into the center of the cake is removed and comes clean, remove from the oven. Cool in the pan for 15 minutes, then remove from the pan. Chill in refrigerator for an hour once cooled.

9. TO MAKE THE ICING: In a large bowl, beat the first cup of sugar with the cream cheese using a wooden spoon. Once you reach a paste, add the remaining sugar along with the lemon juice and zest. Beat vigorously to combine. Refrigerate at least a half hour. Ice all over the top of the cold cake, slice into 9 portions and serve.

1. Tilting the cake from the cooling rack onto a plate and then back prevents the cake from forming lines while cooling.

    ....

2. The icing needs to be refrigerated for at least $1/2$ hour before spreading it onto a chilled cold cake, which is not the same as a cool cake.

Orange and Lemon Cake

A seam of bright yellow lemon curd holds together layers of this orange and lemon cake with the hidden addition of grated squash for texture and fat replacement. The orange icing keeps the whole thing from floating straight up to heaven, where your first bite will surely transport you.

SERVES 10
Calories per serving: 222

For the cake:
3   large eggs
1/2 cup sugar
2   cups peeled butternut squash, finely grated
1   cup self-rising flour
1 1/4 cups finely ground almonds
1   teaspoon baking soda
1/4 teaspoon salt
2   oranges
2   lemons

For the middle:
3   tablespoons store-bought lemon curd

For the icing:
3/4 cup confectioners' sugar, sifted
2   tablespoons butter, at room temperature
2   tablespoons fresh orange juice

1. **PREHEAT** the oven to 350 degrees.

2. **GREASE** the base and sides of two 7-inch spring form pans with a little vegetable oil. Place a circle of baking paper into the bottom of the tins and grease again.

3. **IN A LARGE MIXING BOWL,** using a handheld or standing mixer, beat the eggs and the sugar for a full 3 minutes until pale and light. Add the grated butternut squash and mix until well combined.

4. **ZEST** the oranges and lemons with a microplane and add to the flour, ground almonds, baking soda, and salt. Whisk to combine the mixture.

5. **DIVIDE** the batter between the prepared pans and bake for 30 minutes.

6. WHILE THE CAKES ARE COOKING, MAKE THE ICING: Beat the softened butter with the sugar using the back of a wooden spoon until it has the consistency of a stiff paste. Add the orange juice and beat again to combine and smooth. Refrigerate until needed.

7. COOL the cake in the pan for 10 minutes. Run a knife all around the edge of both cakes.

8. UNMOLD the cakes onto a wire rack and remove the paper on the base. Flip them back onto their bases again so that they can cool right side up on the wire rack and avoid getting any lines.

9. CHILL the cakes in the refrigerator for 20 minutes.

10. TOP one layer of cake with lemon curd, top with other cake layer.

11. SPREAD the icing over the top of the cake and decorate with a little orange and lemon zest.

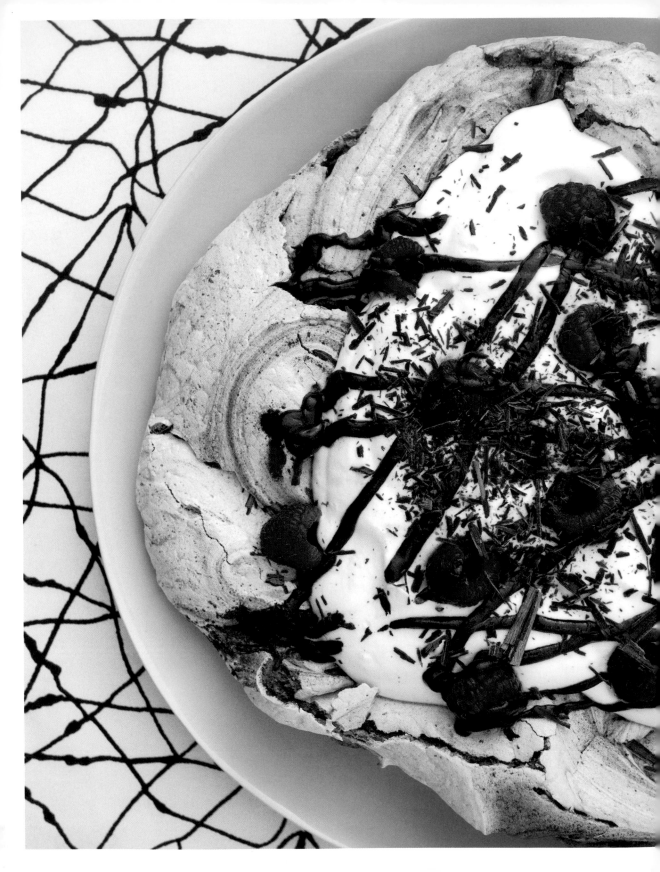

Chocolate Pavlova

It's like tasting a sweet cloud when you grab a forkful of this lighter-than-air dessert, dolloped with cream, raspberries, or your favorite berries such as blackberries or strawberries.

SERVES 6
Calories per serving: 337

For the pavlova:
4 egg whites
¼ teaspoon salt
1 cup sugar
½ teaspoon lemon juice
1 tablespoon cocoa powder

For the topping:
1 cup whipping cream
1 cup fresh raspberries
¼ cup shaved dark chocolate
¼ cup melted chocolate for drizzling

1. **PREHEAT** the oven to 300 degrees and line a baking sheet with parchment paper.

2. **WHISK** the egg whites and salt on high speed until they hold their shape. Add the sugar gradually until the mixture stands in firm peaks. Add the lemon juice and whisk just to incorporate. Sift the cocoa powder into a small corner of the bowl and lightly fold it into the meringue using a plastic spatula. Do not overmix or you will lose the rippled effect. Pour the meringue onto the parchment-lined sheet pan in an oval shape, roughly 3-inches by 5-inches and 2-inches high. Place into the bottom of the oven and bake for 1 hour and 15 minutes.

3. **SWITCH OFF** the oven without opening the door and leave the pavlova in the turned-off oven for one hour. Remove and set aside.

4. **FOR THE TOPPING:** Whisk the whipping cream into semi-stiff peaks and spoon on top of the pavlova. Sprinkle with raspberries and shaved chocolate before serving. Finish with drizzled chocolate.

Tips

1. When mixing meringue, make sure your bowl and beaters are completely clean. Fat will deflate the meringue.

2. Pavlova is easiest to cut and serve with a serrated knife.

3. To ensure a crisp outside and a gooey inside, do not open the oven door during baking.

Chocolate and Raspberry Roulade with Raspberry Sauce

Tender chocolate cake gets invited to a rocking raspberry party in this fruity dessert. Filled, rolled, and topped with a sweet raspberry sauce, we love the way it goes with tea and caps off a meal.

SERVES 9
Calories per serving, roulade: 190
Calories per serving, raspberry sauce: 26

For the roulade:
Confectioners' sugar, for dusting the pan
4   large eggs, separated
½   cup sugar
¼   teaspoon salt
3   tablespoons Dutch-process cocoa powder, sifted, plus more for serving
¾   cup peeled and finely grated carrots
¾   cup self-rising flour, sifted

For the filling:
¾   cup heavy cream
2   tablespoons confectioners' sugar, sifted
1   teaspoon vanilla extract
1   cup raspberries

For the raspberry sauce:
1½ cups raspberries
⅓   cup confectioners' sugar
¼   cup water

1   9-by-13-inch jelly roll pan
Parchment paper, cut to size

1. **PREHEAT** oven to 375 degrees.

2. **CUT** a piece of parchment paper to the size of the jelly roll pan and dust with some sifted confectioners' sugar. Set aside.

3. **REMOVE** 2 tablespoons of sugar and add to a bowl with egg whites, along with the salt. Using a handheld or standing mixer, whip the egg whites until stiff peaks form, about 5 minutes. Take care not to over-mix as the egg whites will become grainy. Set aside.

(continued)

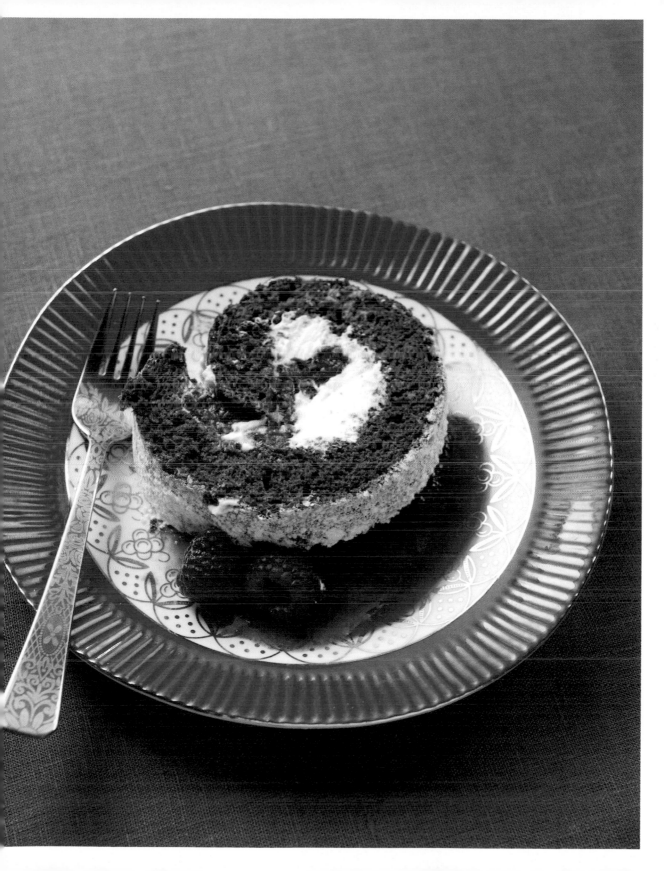

4. **ADD** the remaining sugar to the egg yolks and whisk about 3 minutes, until it is pale and fluffy and holds a ribbon trail when you lift the blades. Add the sifted cocoa powder to the yolk/sugar mixture one tablespoon at a time, whisking it until fully incorporated before adding the next. Once all the cocoa powder is well combined, add the grated carrots and mix well to incorporate.

5. **USING A RUBBER SPATULA,** fold the egg white mixture, one-third at a time, into the yolk mixture, taking care not to deflate the mix. Add the sifted flour into the mixture as you add the last third of the egg whites. Fold as before until all the elements are well combined with no pockets of flour left.

6. **POUR** the batter into the center of the jelly roll pan and tilt it to spread the batter evenly all over the pan, making sure it goes all the way into the corners. Do not pat or knock on the pan as this will deflate the batter. Bake for 10 minutes.

7. **WHILE THE CAKE IS BAKING,** make the filling. Using a handheld or standing mixer, beat the heavy cream for about 30 seconds. Add the confectioners' sugar and vanilla extract and continue to beat until you get stiff peaks. Once ready, refrigerate until needed.

8. **TO ASSEMBLE THE CAKE,** lay a clean kitchen towel on a flat, even surface and place a piece of parchment paper the size of the cake on top of the towel. Once the cake is cooked, working quickly, remove it from the oven and run a paring knife along the edges of the jelly roll pan to help unmold the cake. Take the cake from the edges and flip it onto the parchment paper set on top of the kitchen towel. Peel off the parchment paper.

9. **STARTING** at one end of the towel, roll the cake into a cigar shape, rolling it tightly into a classic jelly roll shape. Continue rolling until the cake is rolled and tucked inside the kitchen towel. Let it stand for 15 to 20 minutes to cool and semi-set in a snail shape while you make the raspberry sauce.

10. **TO MAKE THE RASPBERRY SAUCE:** Add the raspberries, confectioners' sugar and water to a nonstick sauté pan and cook over medium heat, until the raspberries begin to break down and become liquid. Let simmer for about 5 minutes and strain through a sieve into a small saucepan and reduce until thick and syrupy.

11. **ONCE THE CAKE HAS COOLED,** unroll it from the kitchen towel and remove the parchment paper. Spread the whipped cream evenly over the interior of the cake and sprinkle the raspberries. Roll the roulade snugly once again, making sure to tuck in the raspberries as you go along. It may seem like not all of them will fit, but continue to tuck the fruits in generously as you go and they will. Place the roulade on a tray or platter and sprinkle some confectioners' sugar over it. Refrigerate until ready to serve, at least 30 minutes.

12. **TO SERVE,** cut the roll into nine slices and serve with some raspberry sauce.

Vanilla and Strawberry Sponge Cake

The yin and yang of strawberry and vanilla play out on a sweet sponge cake stage. It's a fresh light sweet you'll find a good reason to linger over.

SERVES 10
Calories per serving: 314

For the cake:
1½ cups self-rising flour
1   cup finely ground almonds
1   teaspoon baking soda
3   large eggs
1   cup sugar
     Zest of ½ lemon
1   vanilla bean, split lengthways with seeds scraped out and reserved
2½ cups zucchini, peeled and finely grated
¼   teaspoon salt

For the filling:
10   strawberries, washed and hulled
4   tablespoons of icing (recipe below)

For the icing:
2   tablespoons butter, cut into small cubes and at room temperature
1½ cups confectioners' sugar
1   teaspoon vanilla extract
2   tablespoons heavy cream
8   washed strawberries, halved

1. **PREHEAT** the oven to 350 degrees.

2. **USING A PASTRY BRUSH,** lightly oil the base and sides of two 7 x 2-inch high springform cake pans. Line the bottoms with parchment paper and brush again with a little more oil.

3. **COMBINE** the flour, ground almonds, baking soda, and salt in a small bowl.

4. **USING A HANDHELD OR STANDING MIXER,** whisk the eggs, sugar, lemon zest, and scraped out vanilla seeds until light and fluffy.

5. **ADD** the grated zucchini and whisk to incorporate.

6. **WHISK** in the dry ingredients until they are just combined.

7. **DIVIDE** this mixture between the two springform pans and bake for 30 minutes.

8. COOL on a wire rack while you make the icing.

9. TO MAKE THE ICING, using a handheld or standing mixer, beat the butter until it is softened and pale. Add the sugar a spoonful at a time to form a creamy paste. Add the cream and vanilla extract and mix well. Refrigerate for at least 20 minutes before icing.

10. SPREAD a thin layer of icing on the top of one cake. Top with half the strawberries. Flip over the other cake and ice the bottom, then place this icing side down to sandwich the strawberries.

11. ICE the top of the cake and arrange the remaining strawberries on top and serve.

Tip

You can substitute
1 teaspoon vanilla extract
for the vanilla bean.

Cookies and Cream Milkshake

Old time malt shop flavor without the guilt. Slimmed down dairy and pure vanilla extract may fool you into thinking you're sinning when you're really being good.

SERVES 4
Calories per serving: 169

1   pint low-fat chocolate ice cream, slightly softened
2   packages low-calorie chocolate wafers (about 30 total)
⅓   cup 1% milk
1   teaspoon pure vanilla extract

1. IN A BLENDER, place the ice cream, about 30 thin low calorie wafer cookies, and 1% milk. Add the pure vanilla extract and blend until most of the wafers are broken, leaving a few larger chunks. Pour into 4 glasses and enjoy.

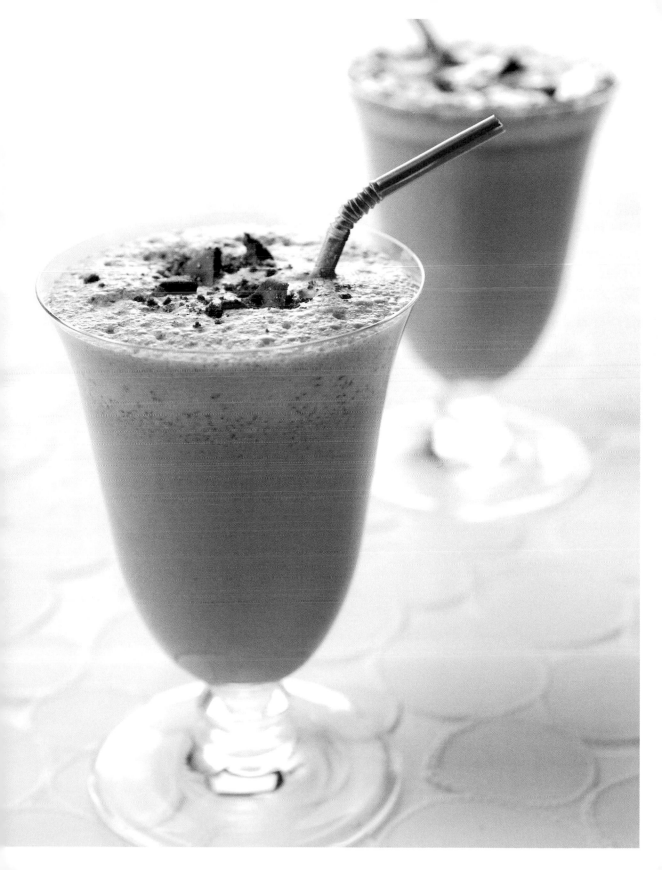

Index

Index

MUFFINS
Banana Chocolate Chip Muffins 86
Lemon and Poppyseed Muffins 88

PASTA
Chicken Tetrazzini 176
Mac and Cheese 167
Pasta Bake with Sausage, Broccoli,
and Beans 112
Pasta Primavera 120
Penne alla "Not-ka" 101
Scrumptious Skinny Spaghetti and
Meatballs 125
Sesame Peanut Noodles 133
Spaghetti Carbonara 157
Spinach and Mushroom Veggie
Lasagna 110
Stuffed Shells 161

PIZZA
Ultimate Sausage Cheese Pizza 137

PORK
Scrumptious Skinny Spaghetti
and Meatballs 125
Sweet and Sour Pork Chops 168

POTATOES
Healthy Potato Skins 115

QUICHE
Mushroom and Spinach Quiche with
Potato Crust 128

RICE
Risotto with Spring Vegetables 181

SALAD
Buffalo Chicken Salad 187
Chicken Caesar Salad 107
Cobb Salad 139

SEAFOOD
Breaded Not Fried Panko-Crusted
Shrimp 147
Mango-Glazed Salmon with Spinach
Salad 143
Portobello Mushroom Tuna Melt 175
Sautéed Tequila Lime Shrimp Tacos
with Mango and Pineapple Salsa
and Spicy Black Beans 140
Spring Rolls with Lemongrass Dipping
Sauce and Cucumber Salad 131
Tuna Salad Rolls with Edamame 188

SOUP
Asian Beef Noodle Soup 192
French Onion Soup 102
Tomato Fennel Soup and Turkey BLT 173

TOFU
Sweet 'N' Spicy Breakfast Hash with
Tofu 82

TURKEY
Sautéed Spinach with Grilled
TurkeySausage and Red Pepper
and Rosemary Corn Bread 148
Scrumptious Skinny Spaghetti and
Meatballs 125
Southwestern Turkey Burgers with
Sweet Potato Fries 99
Tomato Fennel Soup and Turkey BLT
173
Turkey Chili Crunch 122
Turkey Mini-Meatloaves with Roasted
Root Veggies 165

VEGETABLES
Eggplant Stacks 163
Stuffed Portobello Mushrooms 183
Supreme Quesadilla with Poblano
Peppers 158